ESSENTIAL OILS
for HEALING

ESSENTIAL OILS *for* HEALING

OVER 400 ALL-NATURAL RECIPES FOR EVERYDAY AILMENTS

VANNOY GENTLES FITE

with MICHELE GENTLES McDANIEL

and VANNOY LIN REYNOLDS

ST. MARTIN'S GRIFFIN • NEW YORK

ESSENTIAL OILS FOR HEALING.

Copyright © 2016 by Vannoy Gentles Fite, Michele Gentles McDaniel, and Vannoy Lin Reynolds. All rights reserved. Printed in China. For information, address St. Martin's Press, 175 Fifth Avenue, New York, N.Y. 10010.

www.stmartins.com

Designed by Charles Kreloff

The Library of Congress Cataloging-in-Publication Data is available upon request.

ISBN 978-1-250-08260-2 (trade paperback)
ISBN 978-1-250-08261-9 (e-book)

Our books may be purchased in bulk for promotional, educational, or business use. Please contact your local bookseller or the Macmillan Corporate and Premium Sales Department at 1-800-221-7945, extension 5442, or by e-mail at MacmillanSpecialMarkets@macmillan.com.

First Edition: July 2016

10 9 8 7 6 5 4 3 2

To our husbands:
Vance, Jerry, and Jesse

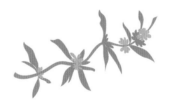

CONTENTS

INTRODUCTION

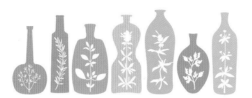

For my family, healing illnesses with essential oils has not always been the case. Once upon a time I relied solely on the medical community and pharmaceuticals for all of my and my family's health care needs. From about the age of three to seven years old my eldest daughter, Lin, suffered from chronic and acute bronchitis. I tried repeatedly to get her help for her condition, but the cure never lasted for very long.

My daughter would start by coughing in the middle of the night, followed by lung congestion, fevers, headaches, fatigue, and a multitude of other respiratory-related symptoms. She would have to miss school and I would lose days of work. When it would get so bad that I feared she had pneumonia, I would take her to a local physician in an attempt to get her well again.

The doctors would always prescribe antibiotics and cough medicine for her. The antibiotics would cause her to develop rashes and the cough medicine often contained codeine, which would turn her into a crazy child. After taking the medications for several days, she would get better . . . for a while. This repeated illness took a huge toll, not only on her, but also on the entire family. I worked at a minimum wage–paying job and didn't have health insurance for anyone in the family. We could not afford to take her to the doctor every other month, pay for the medications, or miss days of work to care for her, but we felt as if we had no choice.

Then I began reading about homeopathy, herbs, essential oils, and home remedies. I studied the materials, talked to people who had used alternative healing methods in their lives, and bought the essential oils and herbs that I had read would put an end to bronchitis. I was adamant that I would take control of her illness and no longer rely solely on pharmaceuticals for her health. This was not a very popular approach in the 1970s and '80s, but I felt that the prescribed medications were not providing a long-term solution.

Soon enough the cycle of bronchitis began again. Lin began to wake up in the dead of night coughing, and her lungs rapidly became congested. I finally decided to make a thyme infusion with honey, and fed it to her by the teaspoon every hour. I made a rub out of eucalyptus essential oil, peppermint essential oil, and olive oil. I applied this to her chest morning and night. I was nervous, and not at all sure I was doing the right thing, even after all of my research. During the first night, she showed marked improvement. I was encouraged by her apparent progress, so I continued her regimen of thyme teas, infusions, and tinctures and the essential oil rub as often as I could. After about three days, her coughing had completely stopped, her lungs were clear of congestion, and she felt like running, playing, and being the active child that she was meant to be. This was the first time in three or four years that I had found an actual cure for my daughter, without just relying on prescription drugs that would mask the symptoms.

I was so overjoyed with my daughter's remarkable recovery that I continued studying essential oils, alternative medicine, and herbs at a frantic pace. I craved any information I could find about homeopathic remedies, alternative healing methods, and herbalism. I was soon incorporating these methods into our daily lives.

My daughter never again got as ill with bronchitis as she had before the essential oils and herbs were applied to her. She did get coughs from time to time, but we always turned to our alternative medicines and cleared her up right away.

There is not an illness in existence for which there isn't a plant that can potentially offer relief. This has become a mantra in our family for the past forty years. While some plants' purposes have yet to be discovered, a multitude of medical benefits have been derived from their essences in the form of essential oils.

People think that *aromatherapy* simply means smelling the essential oils. Nothing could be further from the truth. Although smelling a drop of eucalyptus oil and peppermint oil can clear the sinuses in one breath, there are so many other ways to apply, use, and benefit from essential oils. Various methods of usage include powders, diffusers, rubs, poultices, applied neat (without carrier oil), massage oils, steams, bath additives, inhalers, and countless others, all of which are included in this book.

Having loved essential oils and herbs for most of our lives, we encountered many issues with the books that were available on using them. We wanted a book that is straightforward in its description of the ailments, disorders, and complaints and one that also contains easily accessible recipes. *Essential Oils for Healing* is that book for us and hopefully for you as well.

It lists the subjects in alphabetical order and in a comprehensive, precise way that is easy for the layperson to use. For example, if you are searching for *back pain,* just turn to the Bs and you'll find not just information about back pain, but also a list of all of the essential oils that can potentially help with that condition, any major warnings and contraindications concerning your back pain remedies, and recipes using the essential oils all listed on the same page.

We are passionate about using essential oils in our lives and in the lives of our families. We have experience, knowledge, and an understanding of how essential oils work to provide relief. We have used essential oils to help our friends, our children, and our grandchildren overcome illnesses and complaints for most of their lives. We have each studied, used, and loved essential oils and herbs for several decades.

There is an overwhelming desire today for books that are devoted to the chemical-free and natural-healing lifestyle. Many people don't want to use medications that are actually man-made chemical compounds designed to mimic what essential oils and plants do naturally. Many essential oils can be just as effective—or more effective—in treating illness as man-made chemical drugs, but are much cheaper and, in my opinion, better for you. There is a large movement, not only in the United States but also all over the world, to turn toward homeopathic and alternative medicines. People are buying essential oils at a phenomenal rate; they may not know how to use them, but they want to learn. We're confident this book will provide you with a better understanding of how these natural remedies can be used with facts and recipes that are easy to follow and replicate at home.

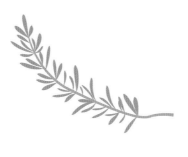

PART 1

BEFORE YOU BEGIN

Ten Tips for Using Essential Oils

Warnings and Contraindications

The 10 Most Popular Essential Oils

Therapeutic Properties and Fun Facts

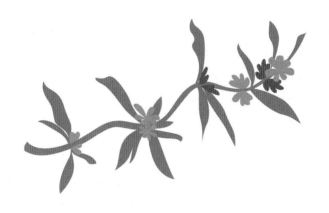

Ten Tips for Using Essential Oils

1. We are not physicians. We do not claim to have any medical training or knowledge pertaining to any of the illnesses in this book or their cures. Essential oils can be used to complement the medical plan prescribed by your health care professional, but do not use any essential oils without first checking with your doctor to ensure it will not harm your condition or interfere with any of your medications. Some medications can be rendered useless when taken alongside certain essential oils, or have other devastating consequences.

2. Ensure that your essential oils are clinical/therapeutic grade. You cannot just use any essential oil that you buy from your local drugstore and expect to get the best benefits from them. Order your oils online if you do not have a good essential oil carrier near you and buy them from a reputable source. I have listed my favorite online sites to purchase essential oils at the back of this book. You can experiment and find the oils that work best for you. Check the reviews and read the labels. You get what you pay for.

3. Never ingest any essential oil that does not state on its label that you can do so. Some brands claim that all of their essential oils are ingestible. I do not recommend accepting this at face value. Do your research first. We only choose two or three essential oils for ingestion in this book, and even those you must ensure are safe by reading the label. If it does not say it is safe to ingest the oil internally, then never ingest it internally.

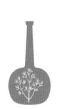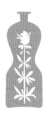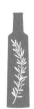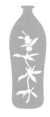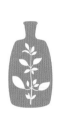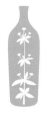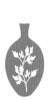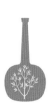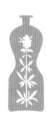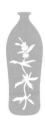

4. Some essential oils can be toxic to children. Never give children any essential oils internally, and never give essential oils to children younger than four years old. Keep lids tightly closed when not in use. Store the bottles in a dark, dry place out of children's reach. I have an old medicine cabinet that my father made years ago. It has sliding doors, tiny long shelves, and is perfect for the storage of many of my essential oils. Be creative!

5. Never touch essential oils to your eyes, ears, reproductive organs, or other sensitive areas. Never apply essential oils to an open wound, cut, or burn. Essential oils are very powerful and strong. You do not want to harm yourself further by getting essential oils into an area they have never been tested on before.

6. Always dilute essential oils with carrier oil, milk, or other liquid unless they are specified to be used undiluted (or "neat"). Carrier oils include olive oil, sesame oil, grapeseed oil, jojoba oil, almond oil, or any neutral oil that you like and works well with your body. When storing your oils or unused portions of mixtures, always use glass containers. I like to use dark-colored amber or green bottles, easily available online. Keeping your oils stored in glass containers in a cool, dark area will prolong the life and effectiveness of your oils.

7. Always perform a patch test before using essential oils on yourself or others. Mix the essential oil in a 1 to 2% dilution for children, elderly, pregnant, or frail individuals: 3 drops of the essential oil mixed with 1 teaspoon of the carrier oil. For typically healthy adults, the ratio would be 3 to 4% dilution: 3 drops of essential oil mixed with ½ teaspoon of carrier oil. Apply one drop of the mixture to your skin and wait 30 minutes to make sure there is not an adverse reaction such as redness, swelling, hives, itching, difficulty breathing, etc. You should ensure that the area does not get wet, as this would dilute the oils and render the test useless. You could cover it with a bandage to protect the area from contamination. Children should be watched closely during a patch test to ensure their safety. Check periodically for 12 to 24 hours. If no redness or any other adverse reaction occurs, then you may assume it is safe for your personal topical usage. If you are allergic to any food made from the herb or plant, then you may assume you are also allergic to the essential oils of the same plant.

8. People who are pregnant, nursing, have high blood pressure or low blood pressure, kidney issues, epilepsy, seizures, asthma, liver issues, heart problems, or any other illness or condition should check with a physician before taking essential oils. Essential oils can adversely affect your medications or your condi-

tion. Read warnings on all essential oils and the "Warnings and Contraindications" section that follows. Heed these warnings seriously.

9. When giving children baths with essential oils, always include 1 tablespoon of milk. This step is not optional for children. It will prevent the oils from adhering to a child's sensitive skin. Always cut the amount of essential oils used in recipes in half when using essential oils on children. Never give a child under the age of four years essential oils.

10. Have fun with your essential oils! Experiment, research, and learn to love these delightful little bottles.

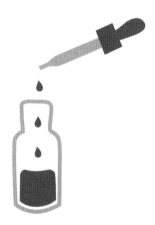

Warnings and Contraindications

If you have any illness or condition, you are responsible for conducting your own research into the essential oils and the effects that they may have on your condition or the way that they may interact with your medications. What follows are the contraindications we discovered in our personal research, but we are not doctors, nor do we work in the medical field in any capacity, and we do not know how essential oils will react with each and every illness, medication, or body type for each individual person. Conduct your own research and perform a patch test before ever using an essential oil. See Tip 7 on page 4 for how to conduct a patch test.

ALOE VERA OIL
No contraindications known by this author.

ANGELICA OIL
Should not be used if you are pregnant or suspect you are pregnant. Angelica essential oil should not be used on small children, diabetics, or persons with epilepsy. This oil should not be used before sun exposure, as it is phototoxic.

ANISE OIL
If you are pregnant or suspect you are pregnant, it is best to avoid anise oil. Do not use anise essential oil for long periods of time or more than twice daily.

ARNICA OIL
Can cause allergies in some people such as rashes, eczema, or hives. Arnica oil must be diluted with carrier oil before applying to skin. Never take arnica oil internally, as it can be toxic. Never apply arnica oil to an open wound.

BASIL OIL
Should never be used in baths, never be used if you are pregnant or suspect you are pregnant, or if you have a seizure disorder. Basil oil should never be used by children and never applied directly to the skin, as it can irritate and burn the skin. Do not use during breastfeeding.

BAY OIL
Do not use for prolonged periods of time.

BENZOIN OIL
Should never be used undiluted. Do not use on children. Be extremely cautious with benzoin oil, as it is very thick and sticky. It will ruin a

diffuser as it will plug up the filter. It will adhere to skin and should be cut drastically with a carrier oil because it will burn the skin.

BERGAMOT OIL

Should never be used directly on the skin or before exposure to sunlight, as it is phototoxic. Should not be used during pregnancy.

BIRCH OIL

Can be very potent to the degree that it can make a person very, very ill. Its painkilling effects are truly amazing, so some people do take a risk to use it for arthritic pain purposes. Never use on children or someone with an illness. Pregnant or breastfeeding women should not take birch oil. If you are ever in a situation where you feel you must use birch oil, reduce it drastically with carrier oil. We have included birch oil in our lists but not in many of our recipes due to its contraindications.

BLACK PEPPER OIL

Can be a skin irritant. Black pepper oil should not be used if you have any kidney issues, as it can be hard on the kidneys.

BLUE CYPRESS OIL

(*See* Cypress oil.)

BORAGE SEED OIL

Do not take while pregnant or nursing. Do not take if you have a liver disorder or are taking blood thinners. Do not take less than 2 weeks before surgery.

CAJUPUT OIL

Should not be used on children. Do not use along with other homeopathic treatments, as it can neutralize their effects. It can be a skin irritant for some people.

CALENDULA OIL

Do not use if pregnant or nursing.

CAMPHOR OIL

Do not apply to broken skin. Do not heat. Children should not take camphor oil.

CARDAMOM OIL

Can be a skin irritant for some people. No other contraindications known by this author.

CARROT SEED OIL

Do not use if pregnant or nursing. Do not use if epileptic.

CASSIA OIL

Very potent; always dilute well with carrier oil.

CEDARWOOD OIL

Should not be used if you are pregnant or suspect that you are pregnant. Children should not use cedarwood oil. Cedarwood oil is a known abortifacient and can cause termination of pregnancy.

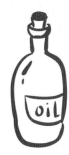

CHAMOMILE OIL

Should not be used if you are nursing, pregnant, suspect you are pregnant, or trying to conceive. Can be a skin irritant. Roman chamomile oil is less irritating than German chamomile oil.

CILANTRO OIL

Should not be used if you are nursing, pregnant, suspect you are pregnant, or trying to conceive. Cilantro oil is not safe if you have any kidney issues.

CINNAMON (BARK) OIL

Should not be used if you are nursing, pregnant, suspect you are pregnant, or trying to conceive. Not to be used on children, in baths or directly on the skin. Cinnamon oil is very strong and can burn the skin. It should be mixed with carrier oil. Do not use during chemotherapy or if you are taking blood thinners.

CITRUS OILS

These oils should not be used before sun exposure as they are phototoxic.

CLARY SAGE OIL

Should not be used if you are nursing, pregnant, suspect you are pregnant, or trying to conceive. Do not mix clary sage oil with alcohol. Do not use clary sage oil if driving. Do not use if you have low blood pressure.

CLEMATIS OIL

Fresh clematis oil is UNSAFE to take by mouth. It can cause colic, diarrhea, and severe irritation to the stomach, intestines, and urinary tract when ingested orally.

CLOVE OIL

Should not be used if you are nursing, pregnant, suspect you are pregnant, or trying to conceive. Clove oil is very strong and can burn the skin. Do not use on children or in baths. Do not diffuse. Do not take with blood thinners.

COMFREY OIL

Should not be used if you are nursing, pregnant, suspect you are pregnant, or trying to conceive. Do not take if you have liver disease or cancer. Never take comfrey oil by mouth or internally in any way.

CORIANDER OIL

Should not be used if you are nursing, pregnant, suspect you are pregnant, or trying to conceive. Coriander oil is not safe if you have any kidney issues.

COSMOS OIL

No contraindications known by this author.

CYPRESS OIL

Should not be used if you are nursing, pregnant, suspect you are pregnant, or trying to conceive. Do not apply to varicose veins.

DILL OIL
No contraindications known by this author.

ECHINACEA OIL
No contraindications known by this author.

EUCALYPTUS OIL
Should be used with caution, as some strong odors can trigger an asthma attack. Should not be used on the face, on children, or with any other medications. Do not use if you suffer from high blood pressure.

EVERLASTING OIL
(*See* Helichrysum oil.)

FENNEL OIL
Should not be used if you are nursing, pregnant, suspect you are pregnant, or trying to conceive. Children or people with illnesses such as epilepsy, any seizure disorder, breast cancer, hormone issues, or kidney problems should not use fennel oil.

FIR OIL
Should not be used if you are nursing, pregnant, suspect you are pregnant, or trying to conceive.

FRANKINCENSE OIL
Should not be used if you are nursing, pregnant, suspect you are pregnant, or trying to conceive.

GARLIC OIL
Should not be used if you are nursing, pregnant, suspect you are pregnant, or trying to conceive.

GERANIUM OIL
Should be avoided if you have hypoglycemia (low blood sugar). Should not be used if you are nursing, pregnant, suspect you are pregnant, or trying to conceive. Can cause insomnia or be a skin irritant for some people.

GINGER OIL
Should not be used on people with very sensitive skin, as it is very strong. Should not be used on people with gallstones or those who are taking blood thinners.

GINGKO BILOBA OIL
No contraindications known by this author.

GINSENG OIL
No contraindications known by this author.

GRAPEFRUIT OIL
Can cause skin irritation. Do not use before sun exposure, as this oil is phototoxic.

HELICHRYSUM (EVERLASTING/IMMORTELLE) OIL
Should not be used if you are nursing, pregnant, suspect you are pregnant, or trying to conceive. Children should not use helichrysum oil. Do not take helichrysum if you are on blood thinners.

HIBISCUS OIL
Should not be used if you are nursing, pregnant, suspect you are pregnant, or trying to conceive.

HOLLY OIL
No contraindications known by this author.

HONEYSUCKLE OIL
No contraindications known by this author.

HYSSOP OIL
Persons with seizure disorder, epilepsy, or high blood pressure should never use hyssop oil. Should not be used if you are nursing, pregnant, suspect you are pregnant, or trying to conceive.

IMMORTELLE OIL
(*See* Helichrysum oil.)

JASMINE OIL
Should not be used if you are nursing, pregnant, suspect you are pregnant, or trying to conceive. Can be used once labor has begun.

JUNIPER BERRY OIL
Should be used with caution, as it is very strong. Should not be used if you are nursing, pregnant, suspect you are pregnant, or trying to conceive. Children and those suffering from kidney issues should not take juniper oil. Juniper oil should never be used for long periods of time.

LAVENDER ESSENTIAL OIL
No contraindications known by this author.

LEMON OIL
Should not be applied directly to the skin. Never use lemon oil before sun exposure, it is phototoxic. Should not be used if you are nursing, pregnant, suspect you are pregnant, or trying to conceive.

LEMON BALM (MELISSA) OIL
Should not be used if you are nursing, pregnant, suspect you are pregnant, or trying to conceive, or have any thyroid issues.

LEMONGRASS OIL
Should not be used if you are nursing, pregnant, suspect you are pregnant, or trying to conceive.

LEMON THYME OIL
Should not be used if you are nursing, pregnant, suspect you are pregnant, or trying to conceive.

LIME OIL
Should not be applied to the skin before sun exposure as it is phototoxic, and should not be used if you are nursing, pregnant, suspect you are pregnant, or trying to conceive.

LINDEN BLOSSOM OIL
No contraindications known by this author.

LOTUS OIL
Should not be used if you are nursing, pregnant, suspect you are pregnant, or trying to conceive.

MANDARIN OIL
This oil should not be used before sun exposure, as it is phototoxic. No other contraindications known by this author.

MANUKA OIL

No contraindications known by this author.

MARJORAM OIL

Should not be used if you are nursing, pregnant, suspect you are pregnant, or trying to conceive. Should not be used during episodes of depression or if you are taking blood thinners.

MELALEUCA OIL

(*See* Tea tree oil.)

MELISSA OIL

(*See* Lemon balm oil.)

MYRRH OIL

Should not be used if you are nursing, pregnant, suspect you are pregnant, or trying to conceive.

MYRTLE OIL

Never take myrtle oil by mouth. Should not be used if you are nursing, pregnant, suspect you are pregnant, or trying to conceive. Unsafe for children or anyone suffering from pulmonary illness or asthma.

NEEM OIL

Should not be used if you are nursing, pregnant, suspect you are pregnant, or trying to conceive. Should not be taken by people with autoimmune disorders, multiple sclerosis, rheumatoid arthritis, or any liver disease. Children should not use neem oil. No one should take neem oil internally.

NEROLI OIL

Can cause dermatitis in some people.

NIAOULI OIL

No contraindications known by this author.

ORANGE OIL

Should not be used before sun exposure, as it is phototoxic.

OREGANO OIL

Should not be used if you are nursing, pregnant, suspect you are pregnant, or trying to conceive. Oregano oil should never be applied directly to the skin, as it can cause burning sensations. Do not use in baths.

OREGON GRAPE ROOT OIL

Should not be used if you are nursing, pregnant, suspect you are pregnant, or trying to conceive.

PALMAROSA OIL

No contraindications known by this author.

PATCHOULI OIL

Should not be taken by people with anorexia nervosa.

PEPPERMINT OIL

Should not be used if you are nursing, pregnant, suspect you are pregnant, or trying to conceive. Never put peppermint oil on neat or in the bath, as it can cause skin irritation. Not to be used by children under four years old. Peppermint oil cancels out any homeopathic remedies, so you should use one or the other.

PERU BALSAM OIL

Should not be used if you are nursing, pregnant, suspect you are pregnant, or trying to conceive. Should never be taken by mouth. Do not take if suffering from any kidney illness. Can cause allergies.

PETITGRAIN OIL

No contraindications known by this author.

PINE OIL

Can be powerful; use in moderation. Pine oil can cause skin irritation. Pine oil should be avoided if you have high blood pressure. Should not be used if you are nursing, pregnant, suspect you are pregnant, or trying to conceive.

PINK GRAPEFRUIT OIL

No contraindications known by this author.

POPPY OIL

No contraindications known by this author.

RAVENSARA OIL

No contraindications known by this author.

ROMAN CHAMOMILE OIL

(*See* Chamomile oil.)

ROSE OIL

Should not be used if you are nursing, pregnant, suspect you are pregnant, or trying to conceive.

ROSEHIP SEED OIL

Should not be used on skin infections, or on people with rosacea.

ROSEMARY OIL

Should not be used if you are nursing, pregnant, suspect you are pregnant, or trying to conceive. Rosemary oil should not be used if you suffer from seizure disorder, epilepsy, or high blood pressure.

SAGE OIL

Never use sage oil if you have high blood pressure or a seizure disorder.

SANDALWOOD OIL

Should not be used if you suffer from kidney issues. Can cause skin sensitivity in some people. Sandalwood oil is getting to be quite rare due to high popularity. Use sparingly to conserve your supply.

SESAME OIL

No contraindications known by this author.

SPEARMINT OIL

Should not be used if you are nursing, pregnant, suspect you are pregnant, or trying to conceive. Never take spearmint oil by mouth.

SPIKENARD OIL

Should not be used if you are nursing, pregnant, suspect you are pregnant, or trying to conceive.

SPRUCE OIL

Do not take if you have asthma or heart problems. Should not be used if you are nursing, pregnant, suspect you are pregnant, or trying to conceive.

ST. JOHN'S WORT OIL

Can have several side effects. Supervise usage and perform a patch test before using. Do not use with other antidepressants. Use caution with this oil before sun exposure, as it can be phototoxic.

SWEET ORANGE OIL

Children should not use large amounts of sweet orange oil.

TANGERINE OIL

Should not be used before sun exposure, as it is phototoxic.

TARRAGON OIL

Should not be used if you are nursing, pregnant, suspect you are pregnant, or trying to conceive.

TEA TREE (MELALEUCA) OIL

Can cause skin rashes and dermatitis in some people. Do not take internally.

THIEVES' OIL

No contraindications known by this author.

THYME OIL

Should not be used if you are nursing, pregnant, suspect you are pregnant, or trying to conceive. Thyme oil should not be used in baths, as it can be a skin irritant. Do not diffuse. People with high blood pressure should never use thyme oil.

TRUMPET VINE OIL

No contraindications known by this author.

VALERIAN OIL

Do not take with other medications. Not enough information known to be assured of its safety during pregnancy or breastfeeding.

VANILLA OIL

No contraindications known by this author.

VETIVER OIL

Should not be taken over prolonged periods of time.

VITAMIN E OIL

Do not take by mouth.

WHEAT GERM OIL

Not to be used by people with celiac disease or gluten sensitivity.

WHITE FIR OIL

No contraindications known by this author.

WILD ORANGE OIL

No contraindications known by this author.

WINTERGREEN OIL

Can be very potent to the degree that it can make

a person very, very ill. Its painkilling effects are great, so some people do take a risk to use it for arthritic pain purposes. Never use on children or on someone with an illness without specific instructions from your physician. When using wintergreen oil cut it drastically with carrier oil. Almost all of the wintergreen essential oils sold today are not true wintergreen oil, but either birch oil or a chemical copy of wintergreen oil. Should not be used if you are nursing, pregnant, suspect you are pregnant, or trying to conceive.

YARROW OIL

Should not be used if you are nursing, pregnant, suspect you are pregnant, or trying to conceive. May cause headaches.

YLANG-YLANG OIL

Should not be used on overly sensitive skin. Should not be used if you are nursing, pregnant, suspect you are pregnant, or trying to conceive. May cause headaches in some people. Do not use if you are taking blood thinners.

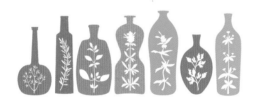

The 10 Most Popular Essential Oils

For anyone just getting into essential oils, first of all, I say, "Welcome!" Second, you may be at a loss for which oils to get and why. This chapter will give you an idea of the most popular and easy-to-use oils on the market, where they came from, and what they are used for today.

The market is flooded with hundreds of types of essential oils, and it can be a little overwhelming. But if you start out with a few of these ten amazing oils, you can rest assured that you will have an oil to meet almost every need. They are the most popular oils for a reason. They work, and they work well—on a number of ailments.

These oils are also the ones used most throughout this book. They each have their own characteristic therapeutic properties and you can quickly become familiar with which oils provide what benefits. Don't be afraid to use your oils!

1. LAVENDER

(Lavandula angustifolia)

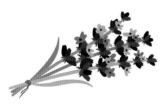

Lavender is one of the most popular essential oils around, recorded as far back as 2500 B.C., beginning with the Egyptians. They incorporated it into their mummification process, and residue of lavender was found in King Tutankhamen's tomb. The Egyptians also used lavender in their perfumes and in incense, which soon spread to the Greeks and the Romans. Mary has been said to have anointed Jesus with lavender oil as a baby and at his death.

Pliny the Elder was said to have recommended lavender for all manner of complaints, from menstrual cramps to headaches. The Greeks and Romans used lavender in their baths, strewn on floors for scent, as an insect deterrent, and in perfumery. In the Middle Ages, lavender was used as an aphrodisiac, and women were said to wear it in their bosoms and place it underneath their beds to attract suitors.

It was during the Renaissance that lavender began to have more of a medicinal reputation.

The "four thieves" developed an herbal wash for themselves and for the items that they stole from graves. After being caught robbing the graves of plague victims, they spilled their secret ingredients, and lavender was given a new life as a protectant against evil and death.

Queen Elizabeth I and Queen Victoria had their castles strewn with the flowers. Hand-maidens were ordered to wash nearly everything in lavender, including the floors, clothing, furniture—even the queen's hair.

During World War I, lavender once again took on a medicinal and protectant role and was used to treat soldiers' wounds after Rene Gattefosse, an early aromatherapist, burned his arm in a lab: thinking quickly and in pain, he placed lavender oil on his arm, which healed the wound quickly without leaving a scar. Word of his findings quickly spread.

Today we use lavender for nearly everything, from perfume to a treatment for depression to an insect repellant. Many people find lavender a useful natural treatment for lice and eczema, too. Lavender has found its way into teas, potpourris, air fresheners, and sunburn treatments. The next time you have gas, a hangover, acne, pain, inflammation, or a minor wound, try a recipe with lavender oil and you will see why it has been a favorite of kings and queens.

2. PEPPERMINT
(Mentha)

Peppermint has been recorded for various uses since at least 1500 B.C. It is believed to have originated in northern Africa and the Mediterranean, as Egyptian medical texts include notes that mint was used for stomach ailments. The herb became so popular that it was used as money: the Pharisees used mint to pay their tithes, and the people used mint to pay their taxes.

In Rome, mint began to be used medicinally when Pliny the Elder suggested that mint was an appetite stimulant. Mint was grown commercially as a digestive aid. In the Middle Ages, mint was used as a tooth cleaner, but it wasn't until the 1700s that medical journals began listing the medicinal properties of mint and its uses: a treatment for venereal diseases, sores, and colds. These Europeans brought peppermint with them to the Americas and discovered that the Native Americans were already using mint medicinally.

Peppermint is thought to be a hybrid between spearmint and water mint. It cannot be spread by seed propagation; it must be spread by the roots. When I have a peppermint plant and tear part of it off to give to someone else to plant, I can't help but think this plant is part of the first peppermint plant that was ever hybridized, split, and shared with another person, in another place and time.

Today, peppermint is used in everything from soaps to toothpaste to medicine. Peppermint is so healing and flavorful that almost everyone can recognize the scent whether it is in their gum, cigarettes, or mouthwash. Peppermint is one of my all-time favorites for almost any ailment or essential oil need.

---

3. ROSE

(Rosa)

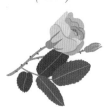

There are fossils all over the world with rose imprints on them, but only above the equator. In 500 B.C., Confucius stated that roses had been planted so prolifically that they threatened to take over farming regions.

The rose probably first bloomed in Persia or eastern Asia, both of which have ancient texts relating to the rose. In Egypt, roses have been found in tombs and were used in religious ceremonies. The ancient Egyptians mixed rose petals with fat and formed them into cones, which they then placed on their heads to eventually melt, perfuming their bodies.

In the tenth century, Persians discovered a way to extract the oil from the rose petals and developed rose water. This was used in many recipes for creams, perfumes, and lotions. It takes about sixty thousand roses to make one ounce of rose oil, making it very expensive, so rose essential oil is often diluted with another, cheaper oil.

Besides sending a dozen of them to a loved one, roses are used today for everything from nervous disorders to massages to tonics. You can find the oil of roses in skin creams, medicine, and perfumes. Rituals are still performed today that include some variation of rose fragrance. Who can resist that beautiful aroma?

4. LEMON

(Citrus limonum)

Before the tenth century, lemons were mostly used as an ornamental plant. The tree is believed to have originated in either China or India. During the Middle Ages, the lemon was transported to Europe, where it was grown as an epilepsy treatment.

Christopher Columbus brought the lemon to the Americas, where it was cultivated and used by the settlers. Later, the Royal Navy used lemons to protect the crew from scurvy due to its high vitamin content. And during the California gold rush, the lemon was used extensively by the miners to protect them from diseases.

Only recently have we begun discovering the beneficial and medicinal uses for the lowly lemon. In Japan they currently run diffusers of lemon essential oils in banks to keep the tellers alert and prevent them from making mistakes.

Lemons are a culinary delight and are fun to use for decorations, but can also be used for everything from natural medicine to cleaning agents. Lemons have come a long way in the last few centuries and their abundance of uses is clearly one of the reasons that lemon essential oil is one of our top ten most popular picks.

5. SANDALWOOD

(Santalum album)

Sandalwood has been around longer than just about any essential oil. It is grown almost exclusively in India, particularly Mysore, and in Pakistan. The Indian government has owned the rights to all of the trees, public and private, since the 1700s, and has enacted strict regulations on the growing, production, and distribution of sandalwood.

Several countries, such as Egypt and China, import sandalwood and use the oil not only for perfumery but for marking graves and in religious ceremonies. Hindus burn sandalwood at funerals, and use the oil to mark the "third eye" in the middle of the forehead. Buddhists use sandalwood in incense burning and in prayer and meditation. In Islam it is applied to graves as a mark of mourning.

Sandalwood is the second most expensive

wood in the world, after African black wood. Sandalwood has a variety of uses today, and is used in everything from anxiety treatments to deodorant to religious ceremonies. Sandalwood is used in treatments for many physical ailments such as cancer, herpes, tumors, and skin issues, but is also used for many mental disorders as well, such as stress, anxiety, and depression.

6. TEA TREE
(Melaleuca alterrifolia)

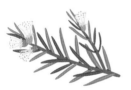

Tea tree is native to Australia and Queensland. The Aborigines have used tea tree to treat their wounds, cuts, and burns for centuries. In the late 1700s, Captain Cook used the leaves of the tea tree to make tea. The Aboriginal people then showed him how to prevent infection using the leaves. He carried this knowledge to Europe, where tea tree was used extensively.

In the 1920s, it was discovered that tea tree actually had over ten times more antibacterial and anti-infectious agents than what was available to the public at that time. In Australia, the soldiers were given bottles of tea tree to carry in their first-aid kits.

Tea tree fell out of favor with the advent of more popular pharmaceuticals until the 1970s, when natural medicine began to make a comeback and large-scale growing was accomplished using new methods. Now, tea tree is used throughout the world as a safe and effective way to heal wounds and prevent infections.

Tea tree is one of the top three most popular essential oils in the world today, due to its ability to help with anything from skin diseases to dandruff and lice. It is even used today to treat certain skin cancers and yeast infections. Tea tree is one of those go-to essential oils that can be used for just about everything.

7. GERANIUM
(Pelargonium)

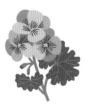

Geranium was first discovered growing in South Africa. In ancient texts, geranium is mentioned as being used throughout Egypt in the treatment of tumors. It was believed to have been transported to Europe in the 1700s; it was used as an ornamental and a table decoration until the 1800s, when its medicinal uses were first discovered.

Geraniums are now grown all over the world, particularly in the warmer climates, as it cannot tolerate frost. It is grown in South Africa, Egypt, Madagascar, and Morocco for the production of essential oils.

Geraniums are the perfect hanging basket plant for your porch, but are also used today for treating many skin conditions from wrinkles to ringworms. It is even used in nerve disorders such as neuralgia and shingles. Geranium oil is included in perfumes, soaps, and insect repellants due to its powerful scent.

8. FRANKINCENSE

(Boswellia)

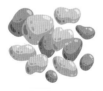

It is said that frankincense was to ancient Arabia as oil is today. The Arabs fiercely guarded their trees and made long, arduous treks through the desert to transport frankincense to trade routes.

The Greeks, Romans, Israelites, and people in ancient Egypt, China, Babylonia, and Assyria all used incense from frankincense in their religious ceremonies and funerals, and many continue to do so today. The Egyptians used frankincense to stuff the body cavities of the deceased in their mummification processes. Many ancient scholars and medical journals sing the praises of frankincense. Pliny the Elder even noted it as an antidote for hemlock poisoning.

Today, the primary countries growing *Boswellia* trees, from which frankincense is derived, are Oman, Somalia, and Ethiopia. The tree bark is tapped, much like maple trees, and the aromatic resin exudes from the tree. This hardened resin is frankincense.

The word *frankincense* may invoke Biblical times, but the oil is very relevant today for its ability to be used in the natural treatment of a myriad of illnesses from rheumatism to Crohn's disease to sore throats. Frankincense is currently being used in treating cancers, stomach disorders, anxiety, eye diseases, and hemorrhoids. But medicine isn't the only use for frankincense oil; it is even being used in soaps, deodorants, toothpaste, insect repellant, and in the culinary world.

9. EUCALYPTUS

(Eucalyptus obliqua)

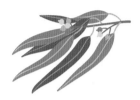

English colonists first discovered eucalyptus in Australia, but the Aborigines had been using it for centuries as a tonic and a cure-all.

Eucalyptus fossils have been found in many countries where it is no longer possible to grow eucalyptus due to climate geographical changes. One fossil found in South America is thought to be over 100 million years old.

Eucalyptus has been traded all over the world because of its overwhelmingly positive medicinal qualities.

Eucalyptus is a great food for koala bears, but is used today in naturally treating everything from skin ailments to pain to asthma. It is even used in the making of musical instruments as well as in candy. It's easy to see why eucalyptus is one of the most popular essential oils in the world today.

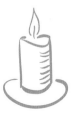

10. HELICHRYSUM

(Immortelle)

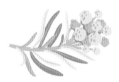

There is not much in the way of history with helichrysum. It originated in the Mediterranean, where it was used pretty much in the same way it is used today, and it has been known to grow in Africa, Spain, Italy, France, and Greece. In ancient Greece it was used as a respiratory medicine.

It was not until as recently as the 1970s that helichrysum was introduced to America. It soon developed a popular following among essential oil users for its medicinal and therapeutic properties and is one of the top essential oils sold today.

A relative newcomer on the market, helichrysum is one of my favorite oils to use for tissue regeneration, circulation, and rheumatism. But those are not its only uses. Helichrysum is used worldwide for its wound, cough, aphrodisiac, and dermatitis healing properties. Some people even use it for hearing loss, bladder disorders, and sunburns. While helichrysum is kind of pricey, it is well worth the money for its powerful healing benefits.

Therapeutic Properties and Fun Facts

Having worked with essential oils for most of our lives, we have uncovered many interesting facts, quirks, and oddities associated with each of the oils used throughout this book, and wanted to include some of the information for you. The therapeutic properties are listed as well so that you can determine which oils are best for your particular needs. See definitions on pp. 46–47.

ALOE VERA OIL

Therapeutic properties: antibacterial, anti-inflammatory, antifungal, antiviral, astringent, laxative, diuretic, immune boosting, antitumor, cicatrisant, cytophylactic, vulnerary, and emollient

It has been a widely held belief that the U.S. government has aloe vera growing underground in bunkers in the event of a thermonuclear war. I don't know if this is true, but I know that it is one of the only true chemical-free cures for radiation burns.

ANGELICA OIL

Therapeutic properties: antispasmodic, carminative, tonic, depurative, diaphoretic, digestive, emmenagogue, expectorant, febrifuge, hepatic, nervine, stimulant, stomachic, diuretic, and tonic

Also known as "holy ghost" and "wild celery," this plant has been used for thousands of years in all types of spiritual rituals designed to bring a person closer to that which is holy. For centuries, angelica has been thought to protect people from evil and the spells of witches. It was grown throughout Europe at monasteries, and has been used for everything from candy making to liquor flavoring.

ANISE OIL

Therapeutic properties: antiepileptic, antihysteric, antirheumatic, antiseptic, antispasmodic, aperient, carminative, cordial, decongestant, digestive, diuretic, expectorant, galactogogue, insecticide, sedative, stimulant, and vermifuge

Anise is grown in the Mediterranean region. In the Middle Ages, it was used in the practice of winemaking.

ARNICA OIL

Therapeutic properties: anti-inflammatory, antibruising, antispasmodic, vulnerary, hair restoration, gastrostimulant, vasodilator, immune stimulant, nervine, and vulnerary

Arnica comes from the sunflower family. It is also known as "mountain tobacco."

BASIL (OCIMUM) OIL

Therapeutic properties: analgesic, antibacterial, antibiotic, antidepressant, anti-infectious, anti-inflammatory, antiseptic, antispasmodic, antiviral, carminative, cephalic, diaphoretic, digestive tonic, emmenagogue, febrifuge, intestinal, nervine, sudorific, tonic, warming

The oil of basil, meaning "king" or "ruler" in Greek, is known in India as a holy oil and has been used as an aphrodisiac for centuries. Thought to be the king of herbs, basil is used extensively in Ayurvedic medicine and can help aid mental fatigue as well as stimulate hair growth and adrenals. A basil plant can grow up to three feet tall.

BAY LAUREL OIL

Therapeutic properties: analgesic, emetic, emmenagogue, nervine, and stimulant

This herb is known by many names: sweet bay, bay, bay laurel, bay tree. Bay is grown in the Mediterranean, and the bay tree is used to make rum.

BENZOIN OIL

Therapeutic properties: antidepressant, anti-inflammatory, antirheumatic, antiseptic, astringent, carminative, cordial, deodorant, disinfectant, diuretic, expectorant, euphoric, relaxant, sedative, vulnerary, and warming

Benzoin has been used in the past to purify surroundings and chase away evil spirits, and has been used for centuries as an incense.

BERGAMOT OIL

Therapeutic properties: analgesic, antibiotic, antidepressant, antiseptic, antispasmodic, cicatrisant, deodorant, digestive, disinfectant, febrifuge, vulnerary, and vermifuge

Bergamot is an herb used in teas all over the world, particularly the famous Earl Grey. I love the smell of bergamot oil and like to use it as a spray, in the bath, and as a powder. It has been said that Christopher Columbus transplanted the tree to several different countries, and it has been used in many countries in rituals to protect people from evil or spells. Bergamot oil is also used in eau de colognes.

BIRCH OIL

Therapeutic properties: analgesic, antiarthritic, antidepressant, anti-inflammatory, antirheumatic, antiseptic, antispasmodic, astringent, disinfectant, depurative, diuretic, febrifuge, germicide, insecticide, tonic, stimulant, and detoxifier

Birch oil has many warnings and contraindications. We have removed it and replaced it with other essential oils in most of our recipes due to its contradictory reputation and its known side effects. It is one of the most powerful remedies for arthritis of all types, but the side effects make it risky to use. When using birch oil, use extreme caution.

BLACK PEPPER OIL

Therapeutic properties: **analgesic, antiarthritic, antibacterial, anticatarrhal, anti-inflammatory, antioxidant, antirheumatic, antispasmodic, aperient, carminative, digestive, diaphoretic, expectorant, and warming**

Black pepper oil is a stimulant and can be used topically for constipation, fatigue, and exhaustion, and to reduce nicotine cravings. Black pepper is grown mainly in India and was traded in the spice wars. It is hot and spicy to the taste. In the Middle Ages black pepper was used in eye ointments.

BLUE CYPRESS OIL

Therapeutic properties: **antibacterial, anti-inflammatory, and antirheumatic**

The oil from the cypress oil tree is blue, hence the name. Blue cypress oil has been used to repel mosquitoes for ages. *Cypress* means "to live forever."

BORAGE SEED OIL

Therapeutic properties: **antirheumatic, cordial, demulcent, emollient, febrifuge, anticatarrhal, antidepressant, anti-inflammatory, antiulcer, and diuretic**

I have loved growing borage, with its little blue flowers, for the past thirty years; it is so dainty and delicate looking. Borage is widely grown in Europe, and its leaves are often included in salads. Borage plants attract bees: we will often watch the bees hanging upside down, drinking from the little flowers, until the bee suddenly falls from its own heavy weight and hits the ground.

CAJEPUT OIL

Therapeutic properties: **analgesic, antineuralgic, antiseptic, antispasmodic, bactericide, carminative, cosmetic, decongestant, emmenagogue, expectorant, febrifuge, stimulant, tonic, sudorific, and vermifuge**

Cajeput comes from the melaleuca (tea tree) tree. It is marketed as BettaFix and used in the treatment of small fish for many of the same purposes that people use it, including fungus, bacterial infections, wounds, ulcers, and tissue damage.

CALENDULA OIL

Therapeutic properties: **antispasmodic, emmenagogue, antipyretic, anti-inflammatory, treatment for sore throat and mouth, vulnerary,** menstrual cramps, cancer, and stomach and duodenal ulcers

Calendula oil is applied to the skin to reduce pain and swelling (inflammation) and to treat poorly healing wounds and leg ulcers. It is also applied topically to the skin for nosebleeds, varicose veins, hemorrhoids, inflammation of the rectum (proctitis), and inflammation of the lining of the eyelid (conjunctivitis). Calendula is derived from the pot marigold. Its most common use is as an ingredient in makeup: it has been said that you should never use a lip balm that doesn't contain calendula oil.

CAMPHOR OIL

Therapeutic properties: anesthetic, antineuralgic, anti-inflammatory, antispasmodic, antiseptic, decongestant, disinfectant, insecticide, nerve pacifier, sedative, and stimulant

Camphor can be used as an embalming fluid.

CARDAMOM OIL

Therapeutic properties: antiemetic, antimicrobial, antiseptic, antispasmodic, aphrodisiac, astringent, digestive, diuretic, stomachic, stimulant

Cardamom oil can be used to neutralize the adverse effects of chemotherapy. Cardamom is grown in the Middle East and is a member of the ginger family. Many Arabs traditionally use cardamom in their coffee. In Scandinavian countries they use cardamom as an ingredient in certain liquors.

CARROT SEED OIL

Therapeutic properties: depurative, diuretic, emmenagogue, vermifuge, and antiseptic

Carrot seed oil is very different and much stronger than carrot oil. Carrot seed oil has long been used by Native Americans in the treatment of worms in the intestinal tract. Carrot seed oil has been used as a remedy in treating hiccups.

CASSIA OIL

Therapeutic properties: antidiarrheal, antidepressant, antiemetic, antigalactogogue, antiviral, antimicrobial, antirheumatic, antiarthritic, astringent, carminative, circulatory, emmenagogue, febrifuge, treatment for menorrhagia, and stimulant

Cassia is the bark of a type of cinnamon tree. Cassia is the most common type of cinnamon sold in America.

CEDARWOOD OIL

Therapeutic properties: antidandruff, antirheumatic, antiseborrhoeic, antiseptic, antispasmodic, astringent, diuretic, emmenagogue, expectorant, fungicide, insecticidal, sedative, and tonic

Cedarwood oil is derived from various conifers, and used to be one of the primary components in paint making as well as in Egyptian embalming practices. Native Americans used cedarwood in their rituals as a purifier, and it was used in ancient days as an antidote to poison. Cedarwood oil has been used all over the world in rituals for centuries, as the word *cedar* means "power." I love the smell of cedarwood oil at Christmastime.

CHAMOMILE OIL

Therapeutic properties: analgesic, antiallergenic, antibiotic, antidepressant, antifungal, anti-infectious, anti-inflammatory, antimicrobial, antineuralgic, antiphlogistic, antiseptic, antispasmodic, bactericide, carminative, cholagogue, cicatrisant, cooling, digestive, emmenagogue, febrifuge, hepatic, nervine, sedative, sudorific, stomachic, tonic, vermifuge, and vulnerary

Chamomile can cool a hot, inflamed area. It can be used as a digestive tonic and for wound healing. It can act as a sedative for the nervous and respiratory system.

German chamomile oil

Therapeutic properties: analgesic, anti-allergenic, antibacterial, anti-inflammatory, antirheumatic, antispasmodic, antibacterial, digestive, fungicidal, and nerve sedative

German chamomile oil is one of the most widely used sleep aids in the world. Its name means "womb," and it is one of the few oils especially safe for children. German chamomile oil is used in some parts of the world to flavor tobacco.

Roman chamomile oil

Therapeutic properties: antispasmodic, treatment for respiratory distress, analgesic, antiseptic, digestive, and nerve sedative

I have grown Roman chamomile for many years. It is a wonderful additive to tea and aids in the sleep process. Roman chamomile comes from the Greek words for "Earth apple" and has long been known in ancient cultures as a Sun God. Roman chamomile was one of the Saxons' nine sacred herbs.

CILANTRO OIL

(*See* Coriander oil.)

CINNAMON OIL

Therapeutic properties: antibacterial, anti-clotting, antifungal, antimicrobial, astringent, carminative, cooling, and stimulating

Cinnamon was first recorded as early as 2000 B.C. Cinnamon oil has been given as gifts to gods and kings and highly prized for ages. Cinnamon is known as a holy spice as it is one of the herbs mentioned in the Bible, but it has an extremely interesting history: the origin of the spice was kept a secret for centuries.

CITRONELLA OIL

Therapeutic properties: antibacterial, antidepressant, fungicidal, insect repellant, vermifuge, and deodorant

Citronella oil repels insects and is used in all sorts of bug-ridding concoctions, from mosquito spray to outdoor candles.

CITRUS OIL

Therapeutic properties: Antitoxic, antiviral, detoxifier, antibacterial, and circulatory regulation

Citrus is great for cleansing metal toxins, such as mercury. There are many types of citrus oil: mandarin, lemon, grapefruit, orange, and the list goes on. Citrus oil is known for its cleansing properties and its bright, refreshing aroma as well as its acidic properties.

CLARY SAGE OIL

Therapeutic properties: anticonvulsive, antidepressant, antispasmodic, antiseptic, aphrodisiac, astringent, bactericidal, carminative, deodorant, digestive, emmenagogue, euphoric, hypotensive, nervine, sedative, stomachic, tonic, and uterine

Clary sage oil used to be known as "clear eye." It was first recorded in 4 B.C. in the Middle Ages; the Egyptians used it as a cure for infertility. It was used in the twelfth through sixteenth centuries to make wine and beer, and also as a remedy for scorpion stings. Clary sage oil can be used to balance hormones, and is a great addition to shampoo to stimulate the scalp and reduce your hair's natural oils.

CLEMATIS OIL

Therapeutic properties: antirheumatic, diuretic, and treatment for blisters, wounds, and ulcers (as a wet dressing in a poultice)

Clematis comes from the buttercup family. Also known as "old man's beard," there are almost three hundred species of clematis. Clematis is one of the flowers used in Bach's flower remedies.

CLOVE OIL

Therapeutic properties: analgesic, antifungal, anti-inflammatory, antimicrobial, antirheumatic, antiseptic, antiviral, aphrodisiac, nervine, stimulant, and immune system stimulant

Clove is smoked in some parts of the world as a cigarette, although clove cigarettes were banned in the United States in 2009. The oldest recognized clove tree in the world is between 350 and 400 years old. In ancient China, people would put cloves in their mouths before speaking with an emperor to kill bad breath germs so as not to offend him. Cloves are stuck into oranges to make aromatic pomanders.

COMFREY OIL

Therapeutic properties: anti-inflammatory, antirheumatic, anticarcinogenic, antitussive, and treatment for menorrhagia

Comfrey is also known as "knit bone," as it was used for ages in the healing of broken bones. Comfrey has been outlawed for internal use in the United States due to its carcinogenic effects when given internally to rats.

CORIANDER OIL

Therapeutic properties: analgesic, aphrodisiac, antifungal, anti-inflammatory, antispasmodic, carminative, depurative, deodorant, digestive, fungicide, lipolytic, sedative, stomachic, vermifuge, and glucose and insulin level stabilizer

Also known as Chinese parsley or cilantro, coriander was found in the tomb of Tutankhamen. It has been said that people are genetically disposed to either hating or loving the flavor of coriander, and that there is no in-between. Coriander seeds are still used to this day to flavor certain liquors. The coriander leaves, cilantro, are widely used in Mexican cuisine.

CYPRESS OIL

Therapeutic properties: anti-infectious, anti-inflammatory, antiparasitic, antirheumatic, antiseptic, antispasmodic, astringent, decongestant, deodorant, diuretic, restorative, vasoconstrictor, and treatment for menopausal symptoms

Cypress originated in Africa, where it was mixed with tobacco and smoked and also used as a disinfectant. In Tibet, cypress oil is used as a purifier and as an incense. The cross that Jesus carried was believed to be made of cypress wood. Cypress is known as the grief herb, and also as the "tree of death."

DILL OIL

Therapeutic properties: antispasmodic, carminative, digestive, disinfectant, galactogogue, sedative, stomachic, and sudorific

In ancient Greece, dill oil was thought to tone muscles and was used by athletes as a body rub to help them shape up for competitions. Dill is used in almost every culture as a culinary ingredient.

ECHINACEA OIL

Therapeutic properties: antibiotic, antiseptic, tonic, antibacterial, depurative, anti-inflammatory, antifungal, antiviral, febrifuge, and immune system booster

Echinacea is also known as "coneflower." Native Americans noticed elk consuming echinacea when they were sick, so the practice of using echinacea as an immune system booster spread throughout the Plains Indians.

EUCALYPTUS OIL

Therapeutic properties: analgesic, antibacterial, antifungal, anti-inflammatory, antimicrobial, antirheumatic, antiseptic, antispasmodic, antiviral, bactericidal, decongestant, deodorant, diuretic, expectorant, mucolytic, and stimulant

Eucalyptus oil can increase circulation, clear the mind, be uplifting, and help reduce negativity. Almost all varities of eucalyptus are native to Australia: more than seven hundred species are from Australia. Some people—me included—are allergic to eucalyptus oil, as the odor can cause a powerful headache.

FENNEL OIL

Therapeutic properties: rubefacient, anti-inflammatory, stimulant, carminative, aromatic, hepatic, expectorant, antiemetic, antiseptic, galactogogue, antispasmodic, digestive, diuretic, diaphoretic, and treatment for bruises

Fennel was used in the past by breastfeeding mothers to increase their milk supply. It was given the name "marathon" in ancient Greece, as it was thought to give strength and long life. Fennel was also used to keep hunger at bay during the Middle Ages. In England, it was thought to ward off evil.

FIR OIL

Therapeutic properties: analgesic, antibacterial, anti-inflammatory, detoxifier, aromatic, antioxidant, and antiseptic

Fir is considered a "middle note" in perfumery.

FRANKINCENSE OIL

Therapeutic properties: analgesic, antiasthmatic, anticarcinogenic, anti-inflammatory, antiseptic, astringent, carminative, cicatrisant, cytophylactic, digestive, disinfectant, diuretic, emmenagogue, expectorant, sedative, tonic, uterine, and vulnerary

Frankincense is known as a "holy herb," as it is one of the herbs mentioned in the Bible, one of the three gifts given to the baby Jesus. At one time, frankincense was thought to be about as valuable as gold, and it has been used in almost every culture to rid evil from the world. Frankincense can grow without soil and has been known to grow straight out of large boulders. It is widely used as incense due to its pleasing aroma.

GARLIC OIL

Therapeutic properties: carminative, rubefacient, stimulant, tonic, antibacterial, hypotensive, antispasmodic, anticatarrhal, anti-inflammatory, antifungal, antimicrobial, antiseptic, antihypertensive, diaphoretic, anticarcinogenic, detoxifier, and expectorant

Garlic has been proven to be a deterrent of colorectal cancer. Garlic was such a popular food additive in ancient days that the Roman slaves held a protest and would not work until it was added back to their diet.

GERANIUM OIL

Therapeutic properties: analgesic, antibacterial, antidepressant, antifungal, anti-inflammatory, antiseptic, astringent, bactericidal, deodorant, hemostatic, cicatrisant, cytophylactic, diuretic, deodorant, styptic, tonic, vermifuge, and vulnerary

Also known as the lemon plant, geranium helps us to keep focus. There are 442 known species of geranium and they come in all types of flavors and aromas. Some species have a long stem and pod that burst open when ripe and spit the seeds a good distance away from the plant. Geranium was used in Britain to ward off evil spirits and negativity.

GINGER OIL

Therapeutic properties: analgesic, antiemetic, antirheumatic, antiseptic, antispasmodic, bactericidal, carminative, cephalic, emmenagogue, expectorant, febrifuge, laxative, rubefacient, stimulant, stomachic, sudorific, and tonic

Ginger makes a good preservative, and is used in cooking throughout the world. Ginger is best known in the United States as a stomach calmer, but it has been known throughout the ages as an aphrodisiac.

GINGKO BILOBA OIL

Therapeutic properties: antiasthmatic, antidepressant, antibiotic, stimulant, circulatory aid, antioxidant, treatment for shock, nervine, treatment for congestion, treatment for infection

This plant is unique, as it has no known relatives in the plant world. Gingko is a living fossil and dates back 270 million years. Gingko trees are some of the oldest living plants on Earth, and the gingko is the national tree of China. After the atomic bomb was dropped on Hiroshima, gingko was one of the few plants to survive and then thrive. It's also great for improving memory.

GINSENG OIL

Therapeutic properties: tonic, vasodilator, anti-inflammatory, stimulant, aphrodisiac, and circulation aid

Ginseng is a billion-dollar-a-year industry. Ginseng oil can reduce herpes outbreaks by 50 percent when taken daily. It's known as an aphrodisiac, brain booster, and a superfood.

GRAPEFRUIT OIL

Therapeutic properties: antidepressant, antiseptic, aperitif, astringent, diuretic, disinfectant, lymphatic, stimulant, and tonic

The ruby red grapefruit is the symbolic fruit of Texas, even though it's been called the "forbidden" fruit. It has been used in different ways to fight obesity because it is thought that grapefruit oil reduces hunger cravings and speeds up the metabolism. Perhaps unsurprisingly, the

United States is the world's largest producer of grapefruit.

HELICHRYSUM OIL

Therapeutic properties: analgesic, anti-allergenic, antibruising, anticoagulant, antidepressant, anti-inflammatory, antimicrobial, antiseptic, antispasmodic, antitussive, antiviral, astringent, cicatrisant, cholagogue, expectorant, fungicidal, hepatic, nervine, and tonic

Helichrysum oil assists with overcoming addiction. Helichrysum is a member of the sunflower family and grows mainly in Africa. It is one of the most expensive essential oils, but well worth it, in my opinion. In some parts of the world, helichrysum is placed on floors to repel bugs and give a pleasing scent when walked upon.

HIBISCUS OIL

Therapeutic properties: antiallergenic, anti-coagulant, antihematomic, anti-inflammatory, antimicrobial, antiphlogistic, antiseptic, anti-tussive, cholagogue, cicatrisant, cytophylactic, diuretic, emollient, expectorant, febrifuge, fun-gicidal, hepatic, mucolytic, nervine, and splenic

Hibiscus is the state flower of Hawaii and the national flower of Haiti and Korea. In these cultures, if a woman wears a hibiscus flower behind her left ear, she is in a relationship; if worn behind the right ear, it indicates she is single and open to a relationship. Hibiscus is made into tea all over the world. It gives a beautiful rosy color and a sweet taste to teas and candy.

HOLLY OIL

Therapeutic properties: digestive, febrifuge, antirheumatic, and emetic

Holly plants are toxic, as are the berries when ingested. Holly is the symbol for truth in many cultures. In the Harry Potter books, holly is the wood used in the titular character's wand.

HONEYSUCKLE OIL

Therapeutic properties: antibacterial, and anti-fungal

There are over 180 species of honeysuckle, and it can become very invasive. When we had a well we wished to cover, we planted honeysuckle and it covered the well beautifully. As a child, I used to pick honeysuckle flowers and drink the sweet nectar that dripped from the bottom of the flower.

HYACINTH OIL

Therapeutic properties: aromatic, calming, and nervine

According to Greek mythology the hyacinth flower sprang from the blood of a man whom the gods admired when he was killed. Hyacinth flowers bloom at Christmastime.

HYSSOP OIL

Therapeutic properties: antimucolytic, antirheumatic, antiseptic, antispasmodic, astringent, carminative, cicatrisant, digestive, diuretic, emenagogue, expectorant, febrifuge, hypertensive, nervine, stimulant, sudorific, tonic, vermifuge, and vulnerary

Beekeepers use hyssop for the bees to produce sweet, rich honey. Hyssop is expensive and hard to find, so I usually order mine online. It has been known to cause seizures in adults and children, so use with extreme caution.

JASMINE OIL

Therapeutic properties: antidepressant, antiseptic, antispasmodic, aphrodisiac, cicatrisant, emmenagogue, expectorant, galactogogue, parturient, sedative, and uterine

Jasmine flowers open only at night. They are so delicate that the flowers cannot be put through the distillation process to make essential oil. Other processes, such as effleurage, are used to extract the aromatic and medicinal benefits. Jasmine is thought to be a powerful aphrodisiac, one of the oils that attracts love, and has been used in many love potions and spells. The flowers must be picked at dawn, before the sun touches them. Jasmine was once used in China to reduce the effects of alcohol or help with a hangover.

JUNIPER BERRY OIL

Therapeutic properties: antirheumatic, antiseptic, antispasmodic, antitoxic, astringent, carminative, circulatory stimulant, diuretic, depurative, sudorific, stomachic, rubefacient, vulnerary, and tonic

Juniper is the ingredient used most often to flavor gin. Native Americans used juniper as a birth control method and in cleansing rituals. It has been used throughout history as a ritual ingredient to protect and as a shield against plagues and diseases, and has been found among ruins in ancient civilizations. In England juniper oil was used to ward off evil and witches.

LAVENDER OIL

Therapeutic properties: analgesic, antibiotic, anticonvulsive, antidepressant, antifungal, anti-infection, anti-inflammatory, antirheumatic, antiseptic, antispasmodic, antivenous, antiviral, bactericidal, cicatrisant, decongestant, deodorant, detoxifier, disinfectant, restorative, sedative, treatment for irritability and nervous tension (great for test anxiety), and tonic

The word *lavender* means "to wash," and hospitals began using lavender in World War I. Its flowers are frequently used in weddings and as cake decorations. In Japan lavender is diffused to help people remain alert on the job. Lavender was said to ward off the evil eye in Europe, and it was one of the first perfumes used in England. A lavender plant produces oil for ten years.

True lavender
(Lavandula angustifolia)

This is the calming lavender essential oil. It can help relieve insomnia, is great for burns, can be applied neat for insect bites and burns, relieves PMS, can be effective against MRSA and tuberculosis, and can be used as a gargle for sore throats or mouth infections (1 to 3 drops in a glass full of water).

Spike lavender
(Lavandula latifolia)

This is the stimulating lavender essential oil. It can be used for chest congestion, sprains, stiff joints, muscular pain, and—my personal favorite—as a flea repellant for dogs! I rub a couple drops in my hands, then pet my dogs all over twice a day when they are in flea-infested areas. I no longer have to give them expensive pills from the vet, and they smell *great*! Do not give to children under the age of ten.

Lavandin
(Lavandula x intermedia)

This is a lavender clone, and is also calming. It is great for use in infections, but do not apply without carrier oil!

LEMON OIL

Therapeutic properties: antispasmodic, astringent, cleanse for liver and gallbladder, detoxifier, tonic, stimulant of white blood cells in body (increasing ability to fight diseases)

In the 1700s, sailors learned that eating lemons reduced their chances of getting scurvy. Now, lemon is one of the most widely used essential oils. Lemon oil can make washing dishes pleasurable: add a few drops to the dishwater. Add it to mop water and kitchen counters. In India, lemon oils are often used as medicine. It can even remove ink stains!

LEMON BALM OIL

(*See* Melissa oil.)

LEMONGRASS OIL

Therapeutic properties: antioxidant, stomachic, sedative, fever reducer, anti-inflammatory, nervine, and immune booster

Lemongrass is commonly planted in gardens to repel insects. It is native to Asia and Australia, and has long been used in Ayurvedic medicine. Now it is used in soap making, perfumery, detergents, and food.

LEMON THYME OIL

Therapeutic properties: decongestant and relaxant

Lemon thyme is my favorite herb to grow. It loves any kind of soil, and when you walk through your garden and brush against it, the scent that fills the air is heavenly. Lemon thyme is also my favorite herb to add to salads. Lemon thyme oil smells like lemon drops, and my grandchildren love to add it to roll-on bottles of carrier oil and use it for some added energy (like they need any)!

LIME OIL

Therapeutic properties: antiseptic, antiviral, aperitif, astringent, bactericidal, disinfectant, febrifuge, hemostatic, restorative, and tonic

Lime originated in Iraq and Persia. The use of lime oil as a protection against scurvy was a British military secret, allowing the navy to remain at sea for longer periods of time.

LINDEN BLOSSOM OIL

Therapeutic properties: diuretic, expectorant, and treatment for high blood pressure

Linden was one of the herbs used to treat women suffering from hysteria. The wood from linden trees is traditionally used to make guitars. It is still used to this day as one of the woods in piano making. Linden blossom honey is thought to be one of the best flavored honeys in the world. Linden blossom is often called "lime tree."

LOTUS OIL

Therapeutic properties: used in chakra work and meditation, calming

Lotus is the national flower of both India and Vietnam and is known as "sacred flower." The lotus flower can live and thrive for over a thousand years, and is used in many paintings, rituals, cooking, literature, and religions. In several countries lotus symbolizes sexual "purity."

MANDARIN OIL

Therapeutic properties: antibacterial, antiseptic, antispasmodic, antiviral, bactericidal, circulatory, cytophylactic, depurative, digestive, expectorant, hepatic, liver protective, nervous relaxant, sedative, stomachic, and tonic

In Chinese medicine, mandarin oil is often used to balance one's *chi*. Mandarin was named after the Chinese officers to whom the fruits were given as tokens of respect, and is thought in many parts of the world to represent abundance and good fortune. The fruit is traditionally placed in Christmas stockings as a treat in several areas of the world. This is a great oil to use for children due to the pleasant aroma.

MANUKA OIL

Therapeutic properties: antiallergenic, antibacterial, antidandruff, antifungal, anti-inflammatory, antihistaminic, an antidote to insect bites and stings, cicatrisant, cytophylactic, deodorant, and nervous relaxant

Manuka was the original "tea tree." It comes from the myrtle family, and its wood is used in making handles for tools and for smoking meats. Parakeets are known to mix the nectar of manuka oil with their saliva and rub it on their feathers to protect them from parasites.

MARJORAM OIL

Therapeutic properties: analgesic, antiseptic, antispasmodic, aphrodisiac, antiviral, bactericidal, carminative, cephalic, cordial, diaphoretic, digestive, diuretic, emmenagogue, expectorant, fungicidal, hypotensive, laxative, nervine, sedative, stomachic, vasodilator, and vulnerary.

Marjoram symbolizes happiness in different areas of the world. It was grown for culinary use by the ancient Egyptians, and Greek newlyweds wore garlands of marjoram for good luck and fortune. In some countries marjoram is used in cooking exactly the same way as oregano. An old saying is that if you keep marjoram near your milk, the milk will not go bad. Good for insomnia blends, aids with cramps, and great to use during cold and flu season.

MELALEUCA OIL

(*See* Tea tree oil.)

MELISSA (LEMON BALM) OIL

Therapeutic properties: antibacterial, antidepressant, antihistaminic, antispasmodic, bactericidal, carminative, cordial, diaphoretic, emmenagogue, febrifuge, hypotensive, nervine, sedative, stomachic, sudorific, and tonic

Melissa is also known as lemon balm. It can be used as an insect repellant, and is a good remedy to treat shock. Melissa oil has been used in many scientific studies related to illnesses such as radiation exposure, Alzheimer's, Graves' disease, and many others, with positive results. Melissa was called "the elixir of life" in the Middle Ages and has been used in winemaking. Melissa oil is very expensive and is often cut with cheaper oils.

MULLEIN OIL

Therapeutic properties: antiseptic, febrifuge, anti-inflammatory, relaxant, and tranquilizer

Native Americans ground the seeds of mullein and used it as fish poison. As the fish would ingest the mullein, paralysis would set in; the fish would then float on top of the water, making them easily accessible to the Native Americans. It has been used as the "drill" in fire lighting, and is smoked like tobacco in many regions in the world.

MYRRH OIL

Therapeutic properties: analgesic, antibacterial, anticatarrhal, antifungal, anti-inflammatory, antimicrobial, antiphlogistic, antiseptic, antispasmodic, astringent, carminative, cicatrisant, circulatory, diaphoretic, expectorant, fungicidal, immune stimulant, mucolytic, purifier, revitalizer, restorative, sedative, stimulant, stomachic, vulnerary, tonic, uplifting, uterine, and vulnerary

Myrrh oil is good for healing mouth sores, and for respiratory health. It is also excellent for healing skin afflictions, and it's great as a natural preservative due to its antimicrobial and antibacterial properties. In Bali, the myrrh seeds are crushed, formed into beads, strung, and worn by women around their hips. Myrrh oil was one of the ingredients used centuries ago to embalm mummies in ancient Egypt. Greek soldiers carried myrrh oil into battle to use in the event of wounds or infections.

MYRTLE OIL

Therapeutic properties: antiseptic, astringent, deodorant, expectorant, and sedative

Myrtle is made into a common alcoholic beverage in Sardinia. The Greek goddess Aphrodite thought that myrtle was a sacred plant and, in some parts of the world, it is used in love and immortality rituals. A sprig of myrtle, plucked from Queen Victoria's wedding bouquet and then planted, continues to give off shoots to this day, and the myrtle is still placed in royal wedding bouquets.

NEEM OIL

Therapeutic properties: anti-inflammatory, detoxifier, and antiparasitic

Neem leaves are used in some parts of the world in cupboards and tins to protect rice and clothing from insects. In India it is eaten as a vegetable, and as a natural toothbrush and toothpaste. Neem has been used to make laundry detergent, natural pesticides, and soap, and has been used in rituals for thousands of years.

NEROLI OIL

Therapeutic properties: antidepressant, antiseptic, antispasmodic, aphrodisiac, bactericidal, cordial, carminative, cicatrisant, cytophylactic, deodorant, disinfectant, digestive, emollient, sedative, and tonic

Good for insomnia, scars, and to treat shock, neroli is derived from the bitter orange oil tree and is known as "orange blossom." Neroli oil is thought to be one of the secret ingredients in Coca-Cola. It is said to take one thousand pounds of neroli blossoms to produce just one pound of the oil. Throughout Europe, during the Victorian era, brides wore neroli blossoms in their hair as a sign of purity.

NIAOULI OIL

Therapeutic properties: analgesic, antirheumatic, antiseptic, bactericidal, balsamic, cicatrisant, decongestant, expectorant, febrifuge, insecticide, stimulant, vermifuge, and vulnerary

Captain Cook named niaouli in 1788. Niaouli comes from the same family as tea tree (melaleuca) oil but is not a skin irritant. It is used in a topical application to the skin before radiation to protect the skin from being burned. It's also good for uterine infections. Niaouli oil comes from an evergreen tree, and the needles resemble rosemary. It is made into a tea in some Middle Eastern countries.

ORANGE OIL

Therapeutic properties: anti-inflammatory, antidepressant, antispasmodic, antiseptic, aphrodisiac, carminative, cholagogue, diuretic, tonic, sedative

Good for flatulence, digestion, stress, and insomnia, there are several flavors and types of orange oil. Orange oil has many uses including as a natural pesticide, cleaning agent, and medicine, and has many culinary and perfumery uses. I have often thought that orange oil is a true pick-me-up. I love to smell it when I am feeling down. Orange oil has been used as tobacco flavoring and as a flavoring for liquors.

OREGANO OIL

Therapeutic properties: analgesic, antiallergenic, antibacterial, antifungal, antioxidant, anti-inflammatory, antiparasitic, antiseptic,

antispasmodic, antitoxic, antiviral, bactericidal, digestive, emmenagogue, fungicidal, stimulant, tonic

Oregano has been known forever as "God's antibiotic" due to its healing properties. We have used oregano tincture, salve, oil, poultices, and compresses for thirty years with our family members to get them over stubborn illnesses.

OREGON GRAPE ROOT OIL

Therapeutic properties: antifungal, antimicrobial, and digestive

Oregon grape root has been used in the making of dyes and in food, jellies, and medicines. This plant grows wild in mountainous regions and is often invasive, overtaking indigenous species of plants.

PALMAROSA OIL

Therapeutic properties: antiseptic, antiviral, bactericide, cytophylactic, digestive, febrifuge, and hydration balm

Palmarosa oil is from the lemongrass family and has been used as an insect repellant and in medicine, cosmetics, and soap. It's often combined with pure rose oil to make rose oil more affordable.

PATCHOULI OIL

Therapeutic properties: antidepressant, anti-inflammatory, antimicrobial, antiphlogistic, antiseptic, aphrodisiac, astringent, bactericidal, cicatrisant, cytophylactic, deodorant, diuretic, febrifuge, fungicide, insecticide, nervine, sedative, and tonic

Patchouli oil is great for the skin and to reduce stress and nervous exhaustion. Incense-loving hippies caused patchouli oil to spike in popularity in the 1970s, and it was used for perfuming ink before the invention of the ballpoint pen. Masters of the Universe action figure Stinkor was manufactured by Mattel using patchouli oil in the plastic mold. It is hard to think of incense without thinking of patchouli, but it's also a very good insect repellant. In centuries past, Chinese merchants used to wrap their silk with patchouli leaves to keep the insects out.

PEPPERMINT OIL

Therapeutic properties: analgesic, anesthetic, antifungal, anti-infectious, anti-inflammatory, antiseptic, antigalactogogue, antiphlogistic, antispasmodic, astringent, carminative, cephalic, cholagogue, cordial, decongestant, digestive, emmenagogue, expectorant, febrifuge, hepatic, invigorating, mucolytic, nervine, stimulant, stomachic, sudorific, vasoconstrictor, and vermifuge

Peppermint oil can be used for nausea, nervousness, vertigo, respiratory problems, digestion, skin disorders, depression, and for headaches and migraines, and as a mosquito or spider repellant. Peppermint is an invasive plant and thought by many to be a nuisance, but pepper-

mint oil has been used for medicine, candy, and gum for years and has recently begun to be used in soap and other cleaning products.

PERU BALSAM OIL

Therapeutic properties: antifungal, antiparasitic, and antiseptic

Many studies have shown Peru balsam oil to be one of the top five allergens when doing a patch test. Peru balsam oil is used as a flavoring in many soft drinks, including Coca-Cola.

PETITGRAIN OIL

Therapeutic properties: antidandruff, antidepressant, antiseptic, antispasmodic, deodorant, nervine, and sedative

Petitgrain oil is closely related to neroli oil and orange oil. Its name means "little fruit." It has been widely used in perfumery.

PINE OIL

Therapeutic properties: analgesic, antirheumatic, decongestant, and deodorant

Pine means "clean" to most people. The smell of pine oil is refreshing, decongesting, and superior to any chemical creation made to mimic its revitalizing aroma. Pine oil is particularly used in men's products such as aftershave and cologne. It has been used throughout the ages during religious ceremonies in many cultures. (I love to use pine oil at Christmastime.) Native Americans once used pine needles as mattress stuffing.

PINK GRAPEFRUIT OIL

Therapeutic properties: antioxidant, energizer, purifier, and tonic

Pink grapefruit is a citrus fruit; many countries refer to it as "shaddock." The essential oil is derived from the peel of the fruit, and it is extremely high in vitamin C.

POPPY OIL

Therapeutic properties: anticarcinogenic, poppy oil with iodine is a treatment for iodine deficiencies such as goiter

Opium and morphine are derived from the poppy. The poppy flower often symbolizes sleep, peace, death, and remembering soldiers who were killed in battle.

RAVENSARA OIL

Therapeutic properties: analgesic, antiallergenic, antibacterial, anti-inflammatory, antimicrobial, antidepressant, antifungal, antiseptic, antispasmodic, antiviral, aphrodisiac, disinfectant, diuretic, expectorant, relaxant, and tonic compound

Ravensara is a very strong antiviral that has been used to treat influenza. It is grown most widely in Madagascar, where its seeds are dispersed by birds that swallow the seeds whole. Ravensara oil is used by some cultures in their rum. It is quickly becoming endangered.

ROSE OIL

Therapeutic properties: antidepressant, antiphlogistic, antiseptic, antispasmodic, antiviral, aphrodisiac, astringent, bactericidal, cholagogue, cicatrisant, depurative, emmenagogue, hemostatic, hepatic, laxative, nervine, and stomachic

Rose essential oil is very expensive, but is still the most widely used oil in the world; it is mainly produced in Bulgaria. Many claim rose oil has the power to make others fall in love with us, and also to help us to love ourselves. Roses were thought by the Romans to stave off the effects of alcohol. They would cover the streets and themselves with rose petals before events. It takes about ten thousand pounds of flowers to produce a single pound of oil. Rose oils are also thought to help people to focus and meditate.

ROSEHIP OIL

Therapeutic properties: vulnerary, antiaging, anticarcinogenic, laxative, diuretic, astringent, anti-inflammatory, and cicatrisant

Rosehip oil has been used for thousands of years by people from widely differing cultures, to reduce scarring and wrinkles. Only thirty years ago studies were completed by various universities that proved the powerful effects of roship oil on aging and scarred skin.

ROSEMARY OIL

Therapeutic properties: analgesic, antibacterial, anti-inflammatory, antirheumatic, antiseptic, astringent, antispasmodic, carminative, decongestant, disinfectant, diuretic, emmenagogue, restorative, stimulant, and tonic

Rosemary is a member of the mint family. In Christianity it was said that the rosemary flowers had been white, but when Mary, mother of Christ, draped her cloak over the plant, the flowers then turned blue. Rosemary oil has long been used in wedding rituals and in love potions. In the sixteenth century, a home that had a rosemary plant was said to be ruled by women, so men began ripping out the rosemary bushes to show that they were the head of the households. Rosemary has long been held to repel witches in the way that garlic repels vampires, and it was used as a preservative all throughout the Middle Ages.

ROSEWOOD OIL

Therapeutic properties: analgesic, antidepressant, antiseptic, aphrodisiac, cephalic, deodorant, and insecticide

Rosewood oil is distilled from the hardwood of the tree. Used mainly for calming and emotional stability, rosewood oil is said to open the heart chakra and allow one to advance spiritually.

SAGE OIL

Therapeutic properties: antibacterial, anticatarrhal, antifungal, antimicrobial, anti-inflammatory, antioxidant, antirheumatic, antiseptic, antispasmodic, cholagogue, choleretic, cicatrisant, depurative, digestive, disinfectant, emmenagogue, expectorant, febrifuge, laxative, and stimulant

It may be better to use clary sage oil, as sage can cause side effects. Sage has been a symbol of wisdom, women's fertility, and protecting one from evil. One of the ingredients in thieves' oil, it has long been used in Ayurvedic medicine.

SANDALWOOD OIL

Therapeutic properties: antifungal, anti-inflammatory, antiseptic, antiphlogistic, antispasmodic, aphrodisiac, astringent, calming, cicatrisant, carminative, decongestant, diuretic, disinfectant, emollient, expectorant, harmonizing, hypotensive, insecticide, memory booster, sedative, and tonic

In the 1700s and 1800s, sandalwood was so highly sought that it was almost sent into extinction. It has been used for centuries in yoga practices and for thousands of years during meditation. Due to its insect repellant nature, sandalwood is often used to make caskets. Various temples that were made of sandalwood in India centuries ago continue to stand today. Egyptians used sandalwood oil in their embalming of mummies. A tree must be at least fifteen years old to get the best fragrance oil from it. Sandalwood is a symbol of purity and is used in many religious rituals and ceremonies throughout the world.

SESAME OIL

Therapeutic properties: anticarcinogenic, anti-inflammatory, antioxidant, and anti-rheumatic

Records from four thousand years ago mention the usage of sesame oils, making it the oldest by far of all essential oils. In some parts of the world, a person who is selfish or of no use is known as a sesame.

SPEARMINT OIL

Therapeutic properties: antiseptic, antispasmodic, carminative, cephalic, emmenagogue, expectorant, insecticide, nervine, restorative, stimulant, and tonic

Spearmint oil is good for reducing fatigue, stress, and nervousness. It can also be used in hypnotherapy to digress one back to childhood. Spearmint is grown in about every country in the world. It is widely used as an ingredient in cooking, teas, medicines, and candies. The name is derived from the leaves, which have a spear shape.

SPIKENARD OIL

Therapeutic properties: antibacterial, anti-fungal, anti-inflammatory, deodorant, laxative, relaxant, sedative, and uterine

Spikenard is one of the holy herbs listed in the Bible. A part of the lavender family, spikenard oil is used in Ayurvedic medicine in India. It was one of the luxury perfumes in ancient Egypt. Spikenard is related to valerian.

SPRUCE OIL

Therapeutic properties: anti-infectious, anti-inflammatory, antispasmodic, expectorant, immune system stimulant, antimicrobial, restorative grounding, and nervine

In Sweden, scientists have dated a spruce tree to be 9,500 years old. Spruce needles can be ingested in times of emergency and used to hydrate people and provide them with vitamin C.

ST. JOHN'S WORT OIL

Therapeutic properties: antiviral, anti-inflammatory, vermifuge, immunostimulant, astringent, antidepressant, cooling, and treatment for burns and stings

St. John's wort is also known as "red oil" due to its deep red color. Many people use this oil as a treatment before and after radiation.

SWEET ORANGE OIL

Therapeutic properties: anticoagulant, antidepressant, anti-inflammatory, antiseptic, antispasmodic, bactericidal, carminative, cholagogue, digestive, diuretic, expectorant, fungicidal, stimulant, stomachic, and tonic

The orange trees that the fruit and oil derived from were first grown in China. Said to be brought to America by Christopher Columbus, orange trees are now grown extensively in warmer regions in the United States.

TANGERINE OIL

Therapeutic properties: antiseptic, antispasmodic, cytophylactic, depurative, sedative, stomachic, tonic, and treatment for stretch marks

Tangerines were named after Tangier, the country thought to be their origin. Tangerines are related to oranges and are interchangeable with mandarins.

TARRAGON OIL

Therapeutic properties: anti-inflammatory, antirheumatic, antiseptic, antispasmodic, aperitif, circulatory agent, digestive, deodorant, emmenagogue, stimulant, and vermifuge

Tarragon oil can be used to stimulate the immune system and for mental stimulation. Tarragon is one of the herbs in French cooking used to make up the popular ingredient *fines herbes*.

But French tarragon is never grown from the seeds of the plant, as they are sterile. It is grown from root propagation.

TEA TREE (MELALEUCA) OIL

Therapeutic properties: antibacterial, antibiotic, antifungal, anti-infectious, anti-inflammatory, antimicrobial, antiparasitic, antiseptic, antiviral, balsamic, cicatrisant, decongestant, expectorant, fungicide, immune stimulant, insecticide, stimulant, sudorific in nature, vasodilator

Tea tree (melaleuca) oil is great for fighting any infection and helps with skin issues such as acne, burns, dandruff (can be used in children's shampoo to repel lice), MRSA, bacterial infections, preventing radiation burns, thrush, vaginal infections, herpes (can use undiluted on sores before bursting), sunburn, wounds, infections, ingrown hair infections, cold sores, and athlete's foot. It has been used during wartime when medicine was difficult to come by. In World War II, soldiers were given tea tree oil to treat themselves in the event of a wound or infection. Australian Aborigines have used tea tree for centuries as medicine. Tea tree (melaleuca) oil has grown in such popularity in this century that the tree is becoming dangerously rare. Tea tree (melaleuca) oil is safe to use neat.

THIEVES' OIL

Therapeutic properties: antibacterial, antiinfectious, antimicrobial, antiviral, immune support, energizing, stimulant, treatment for dental pain, and antiseptic

Thieves' oil is a blend (most commonly made from cinnamon, clove, lavender, eucalyptus, rosemary, and vinegar), dating back to the Middle Ages. It is said that grave robbers used this recipe to protect themselves from the plague. Rosemary needles, lavender flowers, sage leaves, camphor, garlic, and cloves were soaked in vinegar for a few weeks. The strained concoction was said to protect one from a myriad of illnesses and even death. Today we use the essential oils from these plants and mix them with a carrier oil to protect us from a host of unwanted viruses and disease.

THYME OIL

Therapeutic properties: antimicrobial, cephalic, antirheumatic, antiseptic, antispasmodic, bactericidal, bechic, cardiac, carminative, cicatrisant, diuretic, emmenagogue, expectorant, hypertensive, insecticide, stimulant, tonic, and vermifugal

When my daughter was young and had a cough that could not be cured by doctors, I made her thyme infusions, which she drank for several days and then rapidly got over the cough that had plagued her well into a year. Thyme is my favorite of herbs. I love to grow it, heal with it,

cook with it, and eat it in salads. Thyme oil has become one of my favorite essential oils due to its antiseptic properties, and has been used throughout the ages by almost all cultures. Thyme is also good for stimulating the immune system and treating fatigue.

VALERIAN OIL

Therapeutic properties: analgesic, antispasmodic, calming, nervine, stomachic, cicatrisant, stomachic, tranquilizer, and sedative

Valerian flowers attract a wide variety of moths and butterflies. Valerian also acts similar to catnip in attracting cats. The word *valerian* means to be strong and healthy. The new trend in nighttime teas is to add valerian root to chamomile tea to ensure a good night's sleep.

VANILLA OIL

Therapeutic properties: antidepressant, antioxidant, anticarcinogenic, aphrodisiac, febrifuge, relaxant, sedative, and tranquilizer

Vanilla comes from the orchid plant. It is the second most expensive spice in the world. The vanilla sold to tourists in Mexico is actually a mixture of other beans and spices that mimic vanilla closely, but contains coumarin, which has been outlawed for culinary purposes in the United States since 1954. Vanilla was used as a perfume during the Depression.

VETIVER OIL

Therapeutic properties: analgesic, anti-carcinogenic, antidepressant, antioxidant, aphrodisiac, antirheumatic, febrifuge, sedative, and tranquilizer

Vetiver oil is good for relaxing and can be used on the back of the neck (neat) for children with ADHD to aid in concentration and focus. Vetiver is fibrous and has been used in the making of rope. It's also a known pesticide and termite repellant. Vetiver has been used for ages in India as mats for doorways and floors and leaves a fresh scent behind when walked upon. Vetiver is known to protect the soil from erosion. Vetiver oil is used often in Ayurveda.

VITAMIN E OIL

Therapeutic properties: antiaging, anticancer, antioxidant, cicatrisant, ophthalmic, moisturizer for skin

Vitamin E is produced from wheat germ oil, safflower oil, and sunflower oil. It is reported to be one of the best substances you can use for your skin. It is included in just about all skin care products. Vitamin E also acts as a preservative in many recipes.

WHEAT GERM OIL

Therapeutic properties: antiaging, antioxidant

Wheat germ oil is great in cosmetics and as a massage oil. The oil is quickly removed from the wheat during processing, as it speeds up the decomposition of wheat. It is highly prized for its amazing nutritional content, but should be refrigerated after opening, as it will spoil quickly once exposed to light.

WHITE FIR OIL

Therapeutic properties: anticancer, antioxidant, anti-inflammatory, antirheumatic, cardiovascular, antiaging, analgesic, antiseptic, and expectorant

White fir is widely planted in parks in the United States.

WILD BIRCH OIL

Therapeutic properties: anti-inflammatory, antimucolytic, antineuralgic, antirheumatic, antitussive, astringent, carminative, diuretic, emmenagogue, galactagogue, and stimulant

Wild birch oil is commonly used in men's cologne and other fragrance products. Wild birch is commonly used today in making root beer.

WILD ORANGE OIL

Therapeutic properties: antimicrobiotic, antiseptic, antirheumatic, carminative, digestive aid, diuretic, detoxifier, febrifuge, depurative, stomachic, and hypotensive

Wild orange essential oil is said to be very good

for opening the heart, mind, and spirit. This oil is one of the most popular essential oils in the United States due to its uplifting properties and its sweet, strong smell.

WINTERGREEN OIL

Therapeutic properties: analgesic, anodyne, antiarthritic, antirheumatic, antispasmodic, antiseptic, aromatic, astringent, carminative, diuretic, emmenagogue, and stimulant

There is no true wintergreen oil available on the market today. When you buy an essential oil labeled "wintergreen oil," it is either a chemical similar in compounds, or a birch oil derivative.

YARROW OIL

Therapeutic properties: anti-inflammatory, diuretic, antirheumatic, antiseptic, antispasmodic, anticatarrhal, astringent, carminative, cicatrisant, diaphoretic, digestive, hepatic, emmenagogue, expectorant, hemostatic, hypotensive, stomachic, and tonic

In some languages the word for yarrow means "one thousand leaves" and in others it is translated as "little feather" for its soft, feathery stems and flowers. The plant was believed to have kept soldiers from getting infections when they sustained wounds during battle in fields of yarrow. Yarrow was used as a talisman in Scotland to ward off evil. It was thought to be a sacred plant in China and is used to this day to read the I Ching. In Europe it was thought that if a girl slept with yarrow under her pillow, she would then dream of her future husband. Yarrow grows plentifully in roadside ditches all over northeast Texas and in many other areas.

YLANG-YLANG OIL

Therapeutic properties: antidepressant, anti-infectious, antiseborrheic, antiseptic, aphrodisiac, euphoric, hypotensive, nervine, sedative, and tonic

Ylang-ylang oil is a wonderful hormone regulator and is used in massages for its relaxing and sedative properties. Its name means "flower of flowers," and its trees are often called "perfume trees." It's used in the perfume Chanel No. 5. Ylang-ylang flowers are picked only in the early morning, and were once spread on newlyweds' beds in some countries.

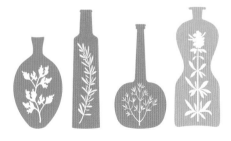

DEFINITIONS

Analgesic – numbs pain

Antiaging – reduces visible signs of aging on skin

Antiallergenic – relieves suffering from allergies

Antibacterial – destroys bacteria, suppressing their ability to reproduce

Antibiotic – fights bacterial infections

Anticarcinogenic – has cancer-fighting properties

Anticatarrhal – removes excess mucous in body, useful in respiratory conditions

Antidandruff – has dandruff-relieving properties

Antidepressant – can help to prevent and alleviate depression

Antiemetic – soothes nausea, relieves vomiting

Antiepileptic – helps reduce or prevent seizures

Antifungal – inhibits growth of fungus (Candida, athlete's foot)

Antihysteric – helps uncontrollable laughing or crying

Anti-infectious – fights infections

Anti-inflammatory – alleviates inflammation, cooling

Antimicrobial – kills microorganisms, inhibits their growth

Antineuralgic – helps reduce sharp, throbbing pain along specific nerves

Antioxidant – counteracts the damaging effects of oxidation

Antiparasitic – treats parasitic diseases

Antiphlogistic – reduces inflammation

Antipyretic – fever reducer

Antirheumatic – prevents and/or relieves rheumatic pain and swelling

Antiseptic – assists in fighting germs/infections

Antispasmodic – relieves spasms and cramps

Antitussive – prevents or relieves cough

Antivenous – prevents clotting

Antiviral – treats viral infection

Aperient – relieves constipation

Aphrodisiac – increases sexual desire

Astringent – contracts and tightens tissue

Bactericide – destructive to bacteria

Balsamic – contains balsam oil

Bechic – cough suppressant

Carminative – prevents or relieves flatulence

Cephalic – relating to the head

Cholagogue – promotes discharge or flow of bile

Cicatrisant – cell-regenerative for skin, healing for scars

Circulatory stimulant – promotes better circulation

Cordial – warm, comforting

Cytophylactic – beneficial for aging and mature skin

Decongestant – reduces nasal mucus production and swelling

Deodorant – prevents body odor

Depurative – cleanses waste and toxins from the body

Detoxifier – removes toxins from body

Diaphoretic – induces perspiration

Digestive – breaks down food in the body

Diuretic – promotes production of urine and rids the body of unneeded water

Emmenagogue – induces menstruation (safe for pregnant women except those with weak or compromised immune systems)

Emollient – softens and soothes the skin

Expectorant – removes excess mucus from the respiratory system

Euphoric – induces feelings of excitement and happiness

Febrifuge – reduces fever

Fungicidal – kills or inhibits fungal spores

Galactagogue – promotes lactation

Hemostatic – helps reduce the flow of blood

Hepatic – beneficial to liver

Hypertension – high blood pressure

Hypotensive – helps to reduce blood pressure

Insecticide – used to kill insects

Intestinal carminative – reduces stomach cramps and colic

Invigorating – incites strength, health, and energy

Lipolytic – assists in the breakdown of fats

Lymphatic – relating to lymph secretion

Menorrhagia – abnormally heavy bleeding during menses

Mucolytic – breaks down mucus, sedative, warming

Nervine – calms nervous tension, soothes nervous system

Ophthalmic – beneficial to eyes

Parturient – about to go into labor

Relaxant – relaxing to the body and mind

Restorative – restores health, strength, or well-being

Rubefacient – topical treatment that causes skin redness and capillaries to dilate, and increases blood flow

Sedative – soothes, calms, induces sedation

Splenic – relating to the spleen

Stimulant – stimulates and increases alertness, increases energy

Stomachic – tones the stomach, increases appetite

Styptic – stops bleeding when applied to wound

Sudorific – induces sweating

Tenosynovitis – inflammation of tendons

Tonic – strengthens and restores vitality to various body parts

Uterine – Having to do with a woman's uterus or womb

Vasoconstrictor – narrows blood vessels

Vasodilator – dilates or opens blood vessels

Vermifuge – destroys parasitic worms

Vulnerary – wound healing

Warming – comforting, induces sense of well-being

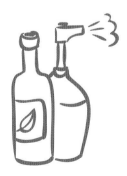

PART 2

AILMENTS AND RECIPES

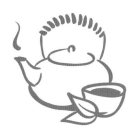

Complete List of Ailments

Essential Oil Remedies

COMPLETE LIST OF AILMENTS

ABDOMINAL PAIN

ABSCESS

ACID REFLUX

ACNE

ADENOIDS

ADHD (ATTENTION DEFICIT-HYPERACTIVITY DISORDER)

AGE SPOTS (LIVER SPOTS)

AGING SKIN

ALLERGIES (SEASONAL)

ANTIBIOTIC MIX

ANTIDEPRESSANTS

ANXIETY

ARTHRITIS

ATHLETE'S FOOT

BACK PAIN

BAD BREATH (HALITOSIS)

BED WETTING (ENURESIS)

BIPOLAR DISORDER

BLEEDING

BLOATING

BOILS

BRONCHITIS

BURNS

CARPAL TUNNEL SYNDROME

CATARRH

CELLULITE

CHAPPED LIPS

CIRCULATION (POOR)

COLDS

COLD SORES

CONCENTRATION

CONGESTION

CONSTIPATION

COUGH

CUTS

DEPRESSION

DERMATITIS

DETOX

DIARRHEA

DIGESTION ISSUES

DRY SKIN

EARACHE

ECZEMA

ENERGY

EXHAUSTION

EYESTRAIN

FATIGUE

FEVER

FLU

FUNGUS

GERMS

HAIR LOSS

HANGOVER

HAY FEVER

HEADACHE

HEARING LOSS

HEARTBURN

HEAT EXHAUSTION

HEMORRHOIDS

HICCUPS

HIGH BLOOD PRESSURE (HYPERTENSION)

HIVES

HORMONE IMBALANCE

HOT FLASHES

IMMUNODEFICIENCY DISORDER

IMPETIGO

INDIGESTION

INFECTION

INFLAMMATION

INSECT BITES/STINGS

INSECT REPELLANT

INSOMNIA

IRRITABLE BOWEL
SYNDROME (IBS)

JET LAG

JOINT PAIN

KNEE INJURY/PAIN

LARYNGITIS

LICE

LOW BLOOD PRESSURE
(HYPOTENSION)

MENOPAUSE

MENSTRUAL CRAMPS

MIGRAINE

MOTION SICKNESS

MUSCLE/LIGAMENT/
TENDON PAIN

MUSCLE SPASM

NAUSEA

NECK PAIN

NERVE PAIN
(NEURALGIA)

NOSEBLEED

OBESITY

OCD (OBSESSIVE
COMPULSIVE DISORDER)

OSTEOARTHRITIS

PANIC ATTACKS

PERIODONTAL DISEASE

PINCHED NERVE

PLANTAR FASCIITIS

PLEURISY

PMS (PREMENSTRUAL
SYNDROME)

POISON IVY/OAK/SUMAC

PROSTATE PROBLEMS

PSORIASIS

PULMONARY CONDITIONS

RASH

RESPIRATORY INFECTION

RESTLESS LEG SYNDROME

RHEUMATOID ARTHRITIS

RINGWORM

ROSACEA

SCABIES

SCARS

SINUSITIS

SKIN TAGS

SLEEP APNEA

SMELL, LOSS OF
(ANOSMIA)

SMOKING, QUITTING

SNORING

SORE THROAT

SPLINTER

SPRAIN

STRESS

STRETCH MARKS

STYE

SUNBURN

TENDONITIS

THYROID DISORDER

TINNITUS

TONSILLITIS

TOOTHACHE

ULCERS
(MOUTH)

VAGINAL ITCH

VARICOSE VEINS

VERTIGO

VIRAL INFECTION

WARTS

WITHDRAWAL
(DRUGS, ALCOHOL,
AND TOBACCO)

WOUNDS

YEAST INFECTION

This chapter lists 136 common complaints, conditions, and ailments in alphabetical order. Each condition is followed by a list of essential oils that have the therapeutic properties needed to heal, help, and relieve your particular conditions. Patch tests are recommended for each essential oil for first-time use to ensure that no ill effects are experienced when using the recipes (see Warnings and Contraindications on page 6).

Each ailment is followed by recipes for that particular complaint or need. The recipes in this book have been used for decades and the plants from which they were derived have been used for these particular conditions for centuries. You may experiment and come up with the ideal recipe for you and your family using the lists of essential oils for each condition.

Most of these recipes include carrier oils to reduce the skin-irritating qualities of the essential oils. Any type of oil that you feel is good for your skin can be used as a carrier oil: jojoba oil, olive oil, rosehip oil, grapeseed oil, coconut oil, vegetable oil, sesame oil, and so on. It is my hope that you have many years of healing with the recipes in this book.

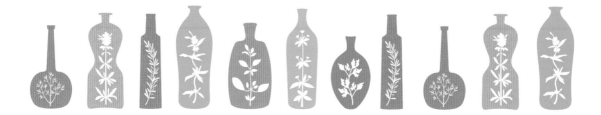

ABDOMINAL PAIN

Pain in the abdomen can range from mild due to gas, virus, menses, or any number of complaints, to severe, as in the case of cancer, appendicitis, or other crises. Food allergies have been a huge culprit for the past couple of decades. With widespread changes to the biological structures of foods, more and more people are becoming sensitive and experiencing abdominal distress. If pain is severe or chronic, seek medical treatment immediately.

Essential Oils: chamomile, calendula, clove, and peppermint

TUMMY MASSAGE OIL

This recipe is good for calming an upset stomach and providing relief to the patient. Calendula oil is an antispasmodic, thereby reducing cramps and spasms. This blend also contains analgesic, anti-inflammatory, antispasmodic, and carminative properties.

YIELD: 3 TO 4 APPLICATIONS

1 drop calendula oil
1 drop clove oil

1 drop peppermint oil
1 ounce carrier oil

Place the essential oils in a small glass jar or container using an eyedropper or the dropper spout included with your essential oils. Pour the carrier oil into the container. Swirl to mix the ingredients. Using your fingertips, apply the oil to the abdominal area and massage lightly into the skin. This can be repeated as needed. Store the unused portion in a jar with a tight-fitting lid, in a cool, dry, dark area, for up to 3 months.

BATH-TIME RELIEVER

Relaxing into a bath loaded with these healing essential oils, stomach muscles calm and cramping subsides. Chamomile oil is an analgesic, thereby numbing pain. This recipe includes oils that have antispasmodic, emmenagogue, and sedative properties. This is a favorite recipe in my family that we have used for many years to bring relief for abdomen and stomach issues.

YIELD: 1 APPLICATION

5 drops chamomile oil
4 drops calendula oil
1 tablespoon carrier oil
*1 tablespoon milk (optional for adults,
    recommended for children)*

Use an eyedropper or the dropper spout that comes with the essential oils to drop the exact number of drops into the bathtub. While the bathwater is running, pour the essential oils and carrier oil into the bath. Make sure that the water is not too hot, as this will cause the essential oils to dissipate. Oftentimes people add one tablespoon of milk to the water; this will cause the essential oils to blend into the water and not float on top. Soak in the water as long as you are comfortable.

ABSCESS

An infection localized to a particular area, inside or outside the body. The point of infection may need to be lanced by a medical professional to rid the body of toxins. Oftentimes the pain can be accompanied by other symptoms such as fever, chills, or fatigue. For thousands of years plants and herbs have been used to reduce the inflammation and ease the pain of external and/or tooth abscesses. More recently, essential oils have been utilized to bring relief to the pain of an abscess and, in some cases, heal it. Seek medical treatment immediately if you suspect you have an abscess.

Essential Oils: echinacea, frankincense, lavender, thieves', lemon, thyme, clove, chamomile, oregano, tea tree (melaleuca), ravensara, and manuka

TOOTH ABSCESS BALL

This is an old, comforting healing remedy that brings about almost instantaneous relief. These oils contain analgesic, antibiotic, anti-infectious, anti-inflammatory, and antiseptic properties, which heal, protect, and clean your aching tooth.

Yield: 1 application

2 drops Roman chamomile oil
1 drop tea tree (melaleuca) oil

Place the drops of essential oil on a cotton ball using an eyedropper or the spout included with your essential oils, being careful to not get the liquid on your fingers. Place the cotton ball on the affected area and let sit for 15 to 30 minutes, or until pain subsides. Repeat throughout the day as needed. The analgesic properties in the essential oils will help with the pain.

EXTERNAL ABSCESS COMPRESS

This recipe has essential oils that are chock-ful of antibacterial, antibiotic, anti-infectious, anti-inflammatory, antimicrobial, and antiseptic components that will numb pain, prevent infection, and kill germs. My husband had a severe facial abscess, and this recipe helped to ease his pain until he could get to a doctor.

YIELD: 1 APPLICATION

1 drop thyme oil
2 drops chamomile oil
2 drops tea tree (melaleuca) oil
1 teaspoon carrier oil

Use gauze, linen, or any comfortable, clean cloth. Drop the ingredients onto the cloth and place over the affected area. Leave on the area until the cloth is cool, 15 to 30 minutes, or until pain subsides. Repeat as needed. Store any unused portion in a container with a tight-fitting lid in the refrigerator for up to 3 days.

MOUTH ABSCESS MOUTHWASH

Manuka oil is an anti-inflammatory oil, which helps to prevent inflammation and assists with the healing of the abscess. Other healing components in this recipe include antibacterial, antibiotic, anti-infectious, antiseptic, and antimicrobial properties.

YIELD: 1 TO 2 APPLICATIONS

1 drop manuka oil

3 drops tea tree (melaleuca) oil
½ cup water

Combine oils and water in a small glass. Put a small amount into your mouth and rapidly swish around. Spit it all out when done. Repeat several times. Do not swallow. Use only essential oils that are clinical grade and state that they are okay to use internally. Store unused portion in a jar with a tight-fitting lid, in a cool, dark area or the refrigerator for 1 day.

ACID REFLUX

For many people, acid reflux is the cause of many sleepless nights. This is the burning, uncomfortable feeling you get when acid from your stomach escapes into your esophagus. Many are tired of the countless over-the-counter medications reputed to end acid reflux, and are turning to more alternative medicines for healing acid reflux and other conditions. Essential oils that are 100 percent pure clinical/therapeutic grade should always be used, especially if taken orally. If acid reflux is severe or chronic, consult a medical professional, as it could be a symptom of something serious.

Essential Oils: frankincense, lemon, peppermint, ginger, chamomile, orange, sandalwood, eucalyptus, and basil

ACID BE GONE DRINK

Lemon essential oil has many therapeutic properties, but the one that works here is the detoxifying agent. Lemon oil rids your body of toxic waste, acid, and germs and will bring healing and relief to you.

Yield: 1 to 2 drinks

1 to 2 drops lemon oil essential oil (make sure the essential oil is ingestible and clinical grade)
8 ounces water

Mix the water and oil in a glass or a jar and drink slowly, as needed. Store unused drink in a jar with a tight-fitting lid in the refrigerator for up to 1 day.

ANTIACID RUB

Frankincense oil has been used for generations to bring a reprieve to the burning and pain of acid reflux. Frankincense is an analgesic and an anti-inflammatory. It also contains sedative properties that will calm and relax your body system, providing instant relief.

Yield: 1 application

3 drops frankincense oil
1 teaspoon carrier oil

In a small jar or container, drip the essential oil, using either an eyedropper or the spout included with your essential oils. Pour in the carrier oil and swirl to mix the oils. Rub the chest and throat lightly with the oils to ensure they are distributed over the skin. Be sure not to get any into eyes or other sensitive areas. Allow the mixture to remain on the skin all day or overnight. If any of the mixture remains, store in a container with a tight-fitting lid in the refrigerator for up to 3 days.

MAKE IT GO AWAY RUB

Chest rubs are one of the best remedies to bring about rapid results, and these essential oils have pain-reducing and healing properties to bring you relief. Peppermint oil is an analgesic, anesthetic, anti-inflammatory, antiseptic, and digestive healing oil.

Yield: 2 to 6 applications

2 drops peppermint oil
2 drops orange oil
1 drop sandalwood oil
1 ounce carrier oil

In a small jar or container, drip the essential oils

using an eyedropper or the spout that came with your essential oils. Pour in the carrier oil and swirl to mix the oils. Rub the chest and throat lightly to ensure the oils are distributed over the skin. Be sure not to get any into eyes or the groin area. Store unused portion in a jar with a tight-fitting lid, in a cool, dark area, for up to 3 months.

ACNE

Acne is a skin condition most often occurring throughout puberty and reoccurring in women during menopause, but anyone can get acne at any time in his or her life, and scarring of the skin can occur if it's not treated. The oil glands under the skin become infected for a multitude of reasons. Plants and herbs have been used for centuries to put an end to acne and to reduce scarring. Be sure to complete an allergy test if it is the first time you are using one of these oils to ensure you are not allergic to them.

Essential Oils: manuka, cedar wood, rosemary, clary sage, petitgrain, eucalyptus, patchouli, frankincense, grapefruit, geranium, palmarosa, juniper berry, bergamot, lavender, tea tree (melaleuca), lemon, German chamomile, lemongrass, benzoin, and sandalwood

ZAP IT!

This recipe is the perfect blend of healing essential oils to use as a preventative for acne. My sister's grandson used it with great results when he suffered with acne in his teenage years. The essential oils in this recipe contain analgesic, antibacterial, and anti-inflammatory properties that will heal your skin and rid you of those unsightly bumps.

YIELD: 25 TO 50 SPRAYS PER 2-OUNCE BOTTLE

5 drops tea tree (melaleuca) oil
3 drops rosemary oil
2 drops lemon oil
2 drops grapefruit oil
4 drops vitamin E oil
2 ounces water

Combine the ingredients in a spray bottle and lightly spray the face or the affected area. Allow to air dry. The essential oils will be absorbed into the skin by contact. Store in the spray bottle in a cool, dark area, for up to 3 months.

JOJOBA IT AWAY!

The jojoba oil works together with the essential oils to rid your skin of outbreaks and protect your skin from damaging elements. These oils include antiseptic, astringent, bactericidal, anti-infectious, anti-inflammatory, and antiviral properties, which bring about speedy healing.

YIELD: 1 MONTH'S SUPPLY

2 drops clary sage oil
2 drop German chamomile oil
2 drop lavender oil
2 drop lemongrass oil
2 drop bergamot oil
2 ounces jojoba oil

In a small jar or container, drip the essential oils using an eyedropper, or the spout that came with your essential oils. Pour in the jojoba oil and swirl to mix the oils. Rub the acne area lightly to ensure that the essential oils are distributed over the skin. Never apply essential oils to the eyes or groin area. Allow the rub to dry and soak into the acne area. Store in a dark bottle with a tight-fitting lid, in a cool, dark area, for up to 3 months.

SLAP IT ON ME BANDAGE

This is spot on for getting rid of that one stubborn pimple overnight when you have something great to do the next day! Analgesic, antibiotic, anti-infectious, anti-inflammatory, detoxifying, and bactericidal properties all work together to bring rapid healing and protect the skin.

YIELD: 1 APPLICATION

1 drop melaleuca (tea tree) oil
1 drop lavender oil
4 drops carrier oil

Mix the ingredients well. Apply a few drops of the mixture to a bandage or a piece of gauze and secure to the acne-affected site. Leave on for several hours or overnight.

ADENOIDS

Adenoids are a mass of tissue behind the nose and above the roof of the mouth. They sometimes swell in young children, making breathing difficult. Adenoids are often removed at the same time the tonsils are taken out. Once the adenoids are removed, breathing usually becomes much easier. Ensure that the essential oils you use (especially with children) are 100 percent pure clinical grade essential oil.

Essential Oils: lemon, cypress, sage, eucalyptus, rosemary, garlic, grapefruit, peppermint, and oregano

RUB THE PAIN AWAY

My youngest grandson had severe adenoid issues before he had them removed. This recipe would bring relief to him at bedtime. These essential oils have analgesic, antibacterial, antiallergenic, anti-inflammatory, detoxifying, anti-infectious, and decongestant properties to help with the pain, swelling, inflammation, and infection. Make sure that there are no allergies, as the throat is a very sensitive area. Complete a patch test before applying to the throat. Use only on children over the age of four.

YIELD: 4 TO 10 APPLICATIONS

2 drops oregano oil
1 drop cypress oil
3 drops lemon oil
1 drop rosemary oil
2 ounces carrier oil

In a small container, drip the essential oils. Pour in the carrier oil and swirl to mix the oils. You can use your fingertips or a cloth to lightly rub the mixture onto the throat area and ensure that the mixture is distributed over the skin. Be sure not to get any in the eyes or sensitive areas. Store the remainder of the mixture in a jar with a tight-fitting lid, in a cool, dark area, for up to 3 months.

SPRAY THAT BAD STUFF AWAY

This is a spray that can bring pain relief for the person suffering from adenoid issues. These essential oils include analgesic, anesthetic, anti-infectious, anti-inflammatory, and antiseptic properties and can reduce pain in the throat area.

YIELD: 25 TO 50 SPRAYS PER 2-OUNCE BOTTLE

1 drop grapefruit oil
1 drop lemon oil
3 drops peppermint oil
2 ounces water

Combine the ingredients in a spray bottle and lightly spray the outer throat area. Be sure your bottle of essential oil states it is okay to take internally and that they are clinical grade. If they are, then you can spray down the throat. Otherwise, only spray the air and neck area. Store in the spray bottle in a cool, dark area, for up to 3 months.

G-G-G-G-G-G-GARGLE

Gargling for me has always proved beneficial, instantly soothing, and pain relieving. A few of the therapeutic properties you can receive in this recipe to help with alleviating pain in the adenoids are anti-inflammatory, analgesic, anesthetic, antiseptic, and antiphlogistic.

YIELD: 1 TO 4 APPLICATIONS

3 drops lemon oil
3 drops peppermint oil
2 ounces water

Mix all the ingredients together in a jar or glass. Be sure that the oils you use are specifically labeled that they can be taken internally and are of clinical grade. Swish a small mouthful back and forth in the mouth, gargle, and then spit it out. Store unused portion in a cool, dark area, or the refrigerator, for up to 1 day.

ADHD

(Attention Deficit Hyperactivity Disorder)

Most children display tendencies of impulsive, overactive, inattentive behaviors. In children diagnosed with ADHD, these symptoms are more severe and occur more often than usual. These symptoms can lead to underachieving in school, issues with behaviors, and difficulties completing tasks. Recently, essential oils have been used to help children with ADHD focus on tasks and exert more control over their behaviors. Essential oils probably won't completely eliminate your child's ADHD, but these recipes may be able to help him or her focus.

Essential Oils: vetiver, lavender, patchouli, cedarwood, melissa, helichrysum, marjoram, clary sage, dill, frankincense, basil, and ylang-ylang

ADHD POWDER

This is a very calming powder to use if you have trouble getting your child to calm down and sleep. And it also smells heavenly! These essential oils contain antidepressant, sedative, and tranquilizing properties that make them beneficial for relaxation.

YIELD: 10 TO 20 APPLICATIONS

4 drops vetiver oil
3 drops lavender oil
3 drops clary sage oil
¼ cup cornstarch

Combine the ingredients very well with a whisk. Pour into a mason jar with holes poked into the lid. Shake the powder inside a pillowcase or under the sheets, and wake up in the morning with renewed energy after a cool, peaceful night's sleep. Store in a jar with a tight-fitting lid, in a cool, dark, dry area, for up to 3 months.

WHOA, BUDDY!

This recipe is great because not only are the essential oils calming, but so is the massage. This recipe can be used on anyone who is having trouble relaxing. I like to use this on a day that I have overworked and my body refuses to believe I am not going to just keep on keeping on! The therapeutic properties that work well together in this recipe are antidepressant, euphoric, hypotensive, nervine, sedative, and tranquilizing.

YIELD: 2 TO 6 APPLICATIONS

4 drops vetiver oil
4 drops clary sage oil
2 drops marjoram oil
1 ounce carrier oil

Mix the ingredients together. Apply 2 drops to the soles of the feet or under the big toe.

Alternatively, in a small container, drip the essential oils. Pour in the carrier oil and swirl to mix the oils. Rub the back and neck area lightly with your fingertips or a cloth dipped into the mixture . Be sure not to get any into the eyes or sensitive areas.

Store unused portion in a jar with a tight-fitting lid, in a cool, dark area, for up to 3 months.

BATH-TIME RELAXER

It's important to add milk to a child's bath that has essential oils. The milk helps to disperse the oils throughout the water so that they won't just float on top of the water and burn the child's skin. Never use essential oils on a child under the age of four. The oils in this mixture have nervine, sedative, tranquilizing, and antidepressant properties. Vetiver oil has shown so much promise recently in helping children with ADHD to focus, relax, and communicate more effectively.

YIELD: 1 APPLICATION

5 drops vetiver oil
5 drops lavender oil
1 tablespoon milk (optional for adults,
*   recommended for children)*
1 tablespoon carrier oil

As the bathwater is running, pour the ingredients into the bath. Make sure that the water is not too hot, as it will cause the essential oils to dissipate. Soak in the water as long as you are comfortable.

PEACEFUL AIR DIFFUSER

This is one of the most calming of all the diffuser recipes. Sometimes, we just need to smell a calming aroma in the air to relax us and pull the plug on our overactive brains. Tranquilizing properties in these oils can bring a sense of calm to even the most hyperactive mind.

YIELD: 1 APPLICATION

4 drops vetiver oil
4 drops lavender oil
Water

Most diffusers come with directions for using essential oils. Add the manufacturer's recommended amount of water and the oils to the diffuser and run your delightful diffuser several times a day to receive the desired effect.

AGE SPOTS
(Liver Spots)

Age spots are caused by the ultraviolet rays our skin is exposed to throughout our lives, especially from sunburns. Essential oils can lighten and in some cases eradicate these age spots. I have recently begun using beneficial essential oils on my age spots, so hopefully before long I will have skin like I did when I was thirty!

Essential Oils: cypress, tangerine, frankincense, Roman chamomile, geranium, ylang-ylang, grapefruit, sandalwood, helichrysum, patchouli, lavender, peppermint, lemon, oregano, and myrrh

AGE SPOT BANDAGE

This recipe is great if you only have one or two spots that you want to eradicate quickly. These essential oils are known to have beneficial properties that will help your skin lighten and blend in with the rest of your glowing looks. The therapeutic properties in these essential oils are, in part, astringent, detoxifying, tonic, stimulating, antibruising, anticoagulant, and cicatrisant.

YIELD: 1 APPLICATION

1 drop helichrysum oil
1 drop oregano oil
1 drop lemon oil
½ teaspoon carrier oil

Mix the ingredients well. Apply a few drops of the mixture to a bandage or a piece of gauze and secure to the affected site. Leave on for several hours or overnight.

If any of the mixture remains, store in a container with a tight-fitting lid in the refrigerator for up to 3 days. If applying to bandage or skin, use a cotton swab or cotton ball to apply to avoid getting your fingertips in the oil.

JESSE'S SPRAY AWAY

I like to spray this on my face every day. It helps keep age spots away, lifts my mood, and keeps me alert. I carry a small bottle in my purse and use it when I start to feel tired. These essential oils are energizing and will keep my skin glowing. With the properties of antiseptic, cicatrisant, tonic, and astringent agents, the age spots don't have a chance.

YIELD: 25 TO 50 SPRAYS PER 2-OUNCE BOTTLE

3 drops geranium oil
2 drops lavender oil
2 drops tangerine oil
2 ounces water

Combine the ingredients in a spray bottle and lightly spray the age spots and the affected area. Allow to air dry. The essential oils will be absorbed into the skin by contact. Store in the spray bottle in a cool, dark area, for up to 3 months.

SOAK THOSE SPOTS

This recipe is really good for those of us who tend to get age spots on our hands and chest. Soaking in a tub is a beauty ritual that does not feel like a chore, but rather like a reward for a really hard day. I like to light a candle and sip a glass of wine while conducting this recipe. It's hard work, but someone has to do it! These essential oils contain astringent, antiseptic, cicatrisant, and restorative properties.

YIELD: 1 APPLICATION

3 drops grapefruit oil
3 drops Roman chamomile oil
3 drops cypress oil
5 drops lavender oil
5 drops ylang-ylang oil
1 tablespoon carrier oil
*1 tablespoon milk (optional for adults,
    recommended for children)*

While the bathwater is running, pour the ingredients into the bath. Make sure that the water is not too hot, or it will cause the essential oils to dissipate. Oftentimes people add 1 tablespoon milk to the water; this will cause the essential oil to blend into the water and not float on top. Soak in the water as long as you are comfortable.

AGING SKIN

Several factors contribute to our skin's ability to hold up over time, including sun exposure, genetics, lifestyle, and diet. There are a million creams and gadgets on the market today to help you overcome the effects of time and sun on your skin. Taking care of your diet, getting plenty of exercise, and limiting your exposure to the sun are the best ways to care for your skin. And always wear sunscreen. Essential oils and herbs have reportedly had great success in turning back the hands of time and have been used for thousands of years by cultures worldwide.

Essential Oils: geranium, rosehip seed, tangerine, carrot seed, lavender, myrrh, neroli, sandalwood, cypress, lemon, rose, frankincense, rosemary, and jasmine

WRINKLE SMOOTHER

This is a very old recipe that was widely used by women before over-the-counter moisturizers. Try it and see how you like the feel and smell of these wonderful fragrances and properties on your skin. Use your favorite lotion and whisk the essential oils into it for a refreshing and healing product. The skin healing prop-erties in this recipe are astringent, cicatrisant, cytophylactic, and circulatory stimulant.

Yield: 2 to 4 applications

2 drops geranium oil
2 drops lavender oil
2 drops rose oil
2 drops myrrh oil
1 ounce unscented lotion

Add your favorite essential oils from the list above to a mild unscented lotion. Apply to the face and neck area with your fingertips or a cloth. Store unused portion in a jar with a tight-fitting lid, in a cool, dark area, for up to 1 month.

FOUNTAIN OF YOUTH

Ahhhh! Now this is a bath! The healing oils soak into your skin and give you that youthful glow that our aging skin loses over time. It also smells wonderful and has so many amazing therapeutic properties. The essential oils in this recipe contain cicatrisant, cytophylactic, and emollient agents to soften, heal, and benefit our skin.

Yield: 1 application

5 drops neroli oil
5 drops geranium oil
5 drops jasmine oil

1 tablespoon carrier oil

1 tablespoon milk (optional for adults,
recommended for children)

As the bathwater is running, pour the ingredients into the bath. Ensure that the water is not too hot, as it will cause the essential oils to dissipate. Oftentimes people add 1 tablespoon milk to the water; this will cause the essential oils to blend into the water and not float on top. Soak in the water as long as you are comfortable.

TIME TO DIFFUSE

This aroma helps us to overcome that tired, aged feeling and grab the essence of youth to energize our spirits and soul. The uplifting properties in this recipe include restorative, sedative, tension relieving, and cytophylactic compounds.

YIELD: 1 APPLICATION

2 drops lavender oil
2 drops jasmine oil
1 drop frankincense oil
1 drop tangerine oil
Water

Most diffusers come with directions for using essential oils. Add the manufacturer's recommended amount of water and the oils to the diffuser and run your delightful diffuser several times a day to receive the desired effect.

ALLERGIES
(Seasonal)

When breathing in something that one is allergic to, responses in our bodies include excess mucus, itchy watery eyes, nasal discharge, general feelings of malaise, and coughing. There are many medications on the market today to help with overcoming seasonal allergies. Essential oils can assist in clearing the bronchial tubes, loosening phlegm, eradicating headaches, increasing energy, and soothing tired muscles.

Essential Oils: lavender, Roman chamomile, yarrow, helichrysum, melissa, peppermint, lemon, thieves', cedarwood, patchouli, lemongrass, valerian, tea tree (melaleuca), spikenard, and basil

BREATHE DEEPLY

I have several small vials of essential oils that I carry in my purse in the event that I, or a family member, have an urgent need to breathe. Lemon and lavender are two of the oils that I carry on a daily basis. Get to know these oils, as they are invaluable. These two can clear the sinuses and relieve seasonal allergy headaches and stuffiness with their anti-inflammatory, decongestant, bactericidal, antibiotic, and analgesic properties.

YIELD: 1 APPLICATION

1 drop lemon oil
1 drop lavender oil

Place the drops of the essential oils onto a handkerchief, a tissue, in the palm of your hand, or into an essential oil inhaler. Cup the essential oils to the nose and inhale the aroma. Repeat several times daily or as needed.

VANCE'S AIR LIGHTENER

When my husband has his seasonal allergy attacks, I quietly fill the diffuser with a couple of these oils and he stops his sniffling and sneezing and soon feels great. The properties in these oils are detoxifying, disinfectant, restorative, bactericidal, decongestant, and detoxifying agents.

YIELD: 1 APPLICATION

3 drops lemon oil
2 drops lavender oil
Water
OR
2 drops tea tree (melaleuca) oil
2 drops lemongrass oil
Water

Most diffusers come with directions for using essential oils. Add the manufacturer's recommended amount of water and the oils to the diffuser and run your refreshing diffuser several times a day to receive the desired effect.

LEVI'S REFRESHING SPRITZER

This spray has a more "manly" smell than Vance's Air Lightener and is perfect for men to use on the sheets and bedding. These essential oils promote sleep and sweet dreams while making breathing a bit easier. The sleep-promoting properties also clear the lungs with their sedative, analgesic, sudorific, nervine, and restorative properties.

YIELD: 25 TO 50 SPRAYS PER 2-OUNCE BOTTLE

2 drops basil oil
2 drops lemongrass oil
1 drop lemon oil
2 ounces water

Combine the ingredients in a spray bottle. Lightly spritz onto the desired area, such as sheets and pillowcases. Allow to air dry. The essential oils will be absorbed by the skin on contact and breathed into the respiratory chambers. Store in the spray bottle in a cool, dark area, for up to 3 months.

ANTIBIOTIC MIX

Essential oils have been ued for centuries to prevent illnesses. These recipes can assist with fighting off infections, provide you with protection, and help prevent contraction of many illnesses.

Essential Oils: thieves', lime, oregano, lemon, frankincense, cinnamon, basil, marjoram, lemongrass, cassia, camphor, lavender, orange, neem, helichrysum, thyme, grapefruit, rosemary, geranium, chamomile, peppermint, eucalyptus, clove, myrrh, clary sage, and tea tree (melaleuca)

CLEAN THAT COUNTER

Keeping germs at bay is a surefire way to prevent viruses from attacking your family. I use this spray to wipe down my "pleather" furniture, doorknobs, and other areas shared by many. Keeping the home clean and germs far away is easy when you are armed with essential oils containing germicidal, fungal, and antiseptic properties such as the ones in this recipe.

Yield: 50 to 100 sprays per 4-ounce bottle

3 drops lemon oil
3 drops orange oil
2 drops cinnamon oil
2 drops grapefruit oil
3 drops tea tree (melaleuca) oil
4 ounces water

Combine the ingredients in a spray bottle and lightly spray the desired area. Allow to air dry. The essential oils will protect the area from germs and help prevent the spread of illnesses. Store in the spray bottle in a cool, dark area, for up to 3 months.

RUB ME HEALTHY

This recipe can be applied to the neck, back, feet, or anywhere you may want some protection. Germs don't stand a chance when these oils are present due to their antiseptic, antiviral, and disinfectant therapeutic properties. These are some great oils to use when flu season is dropping people like flies. Rub this on the family and they will have an iron fence of protection.

Yield: 2 to 6 applications

1 drop cinnamon oil
2 drops oregano oil
2 drops lime oil
1 ounce carrier oil

In a small container, drip the essential oils. Pour in the carrier oil and swirl to mix the oils. Rub the mixture lightly over the desired area, with your fingertips or a cloth, to ensure that the oils are distributed over the skin. You can also pour it into a roll-on bottle and roll onto the desired area. Be sure not to get any into the eyes or sensitive areas. Store unused portion in a jar with a tight-fitting lid in a cool, dark area, for up to 3 months.

THROAT RUB

You know that coworker who coughs without covering their mouth? Instant force field! Protect yourself with God's little germ fighters. I like to just put a dab of this on each morning at certain times of the year. These oils contain antifungal, anti-inflammatory, antimicrobial, antiseptic, and antiviral properties.

YIELD: 2 TO 6 APPLICATIONS

1 drop cinnamon oil
2 drops lemon oil
2 drops lime oil
1 drop eucalyptus oil
1 ounce carrier oil

In a small container, drip the essential oils. Pour in the carrier oil and swirl to mix the oils. Rub the throat and neck area lightly with your fingertips or a cloth dipped into the mixture. You can also pour it into a roll-on bottle and roll onto the desired area. Be sure not to get any into the eyes or sensitive areas. Store unused portion in a jar with a tight-fitting lid in a cool, dark area, for up to 3 months.

ANTI-DEPRESSANTS

Essential oils have been widely used to lift the spirits, they impart joy and feelings of well-being to those suffering from depression, and they can be a wonderful complement to your medical plan. Essential oils may not mix with your medications, so always consult a physician before using. And never take yourself off of antidepressants except under a doctor's care.

Essential Oils: clary sage, chamomile, rosemary, neroli, ylang-ylang, orange, citrus, melissa, lavender, jasmine, geranium, bergamot, tangerine, mandarin, amber, basil, frankincense, red thyme, sandalwood, grapefruit, vetiver, rose, lemon, lime, spearmint, and thyme

DON'T DWELL POWDER

With this aroma drifting around you as you sink into a deep sleep, you won't dwell on the problems that usually keep you awake. This combination of essential oils will soon have you visiting the dreamland of Utopia, instead of the Land of Numb. Some of the therapeutic properties of these oils contain antidepressant, sedative, and aphrodisiac qualities.

YIELD: 10 TO 20 APPLICATIONS

3 drops vetiver oil
3 drops lime oil
3 drops rosemary oil
¼ cup cornstarch

Combine the ingredients very well with a whisk. Pour into a mason jar with holes poked into the lid. Shake the powder inside a pillowcase or under the sheets, and wake up in the morning with renewed energy after a cool, peaceful night's sleep. Store in a jar with a tight-fitting lid, in a cool, dark, dry area, for up to 3 months.

HAPPY BATH TIME

It's hard to be sad when you have jasmine oil and neroli oil surrounding you with their pleasing aromas. These essential oils and their combination work to stimulate the part of your brain that encourages you to be more pleasant and content due to their tonic and aphrodisiac properties.

YIELD: 1 APPLICATION

3 drops neroli oil

3 drops lemon oil
3 drops jasmine oil
2 drops geranium oil
1 tablespoon carrier oil
1 tablespoon milk (optional for adults, recommended for children)

As the bathwater is running, pour the ingredients into the bath. Make sure that the water is not so hot as to cause the essential oils to dissipate. Oftentimes people add 1 tablespoon milk to the water; this will cause the essential oil to blend into the water and not float on top. Soak in the water as long as you are comfortable.

LIFT UP THE AIR

Happy, peaceful memories are bound to happen when you fill the air with this fragrance. Turn that mood around and join the living again with this combination of essential oils. The healing, calming properties of these oils contain antidepressant, restorative, and sedative agents.

YIELD: 1 APPLICATION

3 drops bergamot oil
2 drops lavender oil
2 drops clary sage oil
1 drop ylang-ylang oil
Water

Most diffusers come with directions for using

essential oils. Add the manufacturer's recommended amount of water and the oils to the diffuser and run your delightful diffuser several times a day to receive the desired effect.

MASSAGE THE BLUES AWAY

I mean, really, who can be depressed when receiving a massage with these lovely essential oils? The plants that these essential oils were derived from have been used for thousands of years to ease the suffering of the mind. This recipe contains antidepressant, calming, euphoric, and uplifting properties.

YIELD: 2 TO 6 APPLICATIONS

3 drops clary sage oil
2 drops lemon oil
2 drops frankincense oil
1 ounce carrier oil

Place the essential oils in a small container. Pour in the carrier oil. Swirl to mix the ingredients and use your fingertips or a cloth dipped in the mixture to lightly massage the desired area. Keep the essential oil mixture away from open wounds or sensitive areas. This can be repeated as needed. Store unused portion in a jar with a tight-fitting lid, in a cool, dark area, for up to 3 months.

ANXIETY

Most people have some experience with this feeling caused by stress, fear, or some unknown factor. A person with anxiety often cannot cope normally in a happy manner. Essential oils can help to alleviate fears and worries and bring a person peace, calm, and joy.

Essential Oils: frankincense, marjoram, clary sage, chamomile, juniper, geranium, lavender, peppermint, neroli, jasmine, ylang-ylang, lemon, petitgrain, sandalwood, neroli, cypress, melissa, hyssop, orange, basil, and rose

ANXIETY QUELLING POWDER

This is the perfect nighttime relaxer for those people whose minds go a million miles an hour and won't shut off, or for when you are consumed by real or imagined fears. I love this stuff when it is bill-paying time and I am stressing about money issues. Financial stress is the worst! Therapeutic properties in these essential oils include antidepressant, nervine, and sedative.

YIELD: 10 TO 20 APPLICATIONS

3 drops jasmine oil

3 drops petitgrain oil
3 drops sandalwood oil
¼ cup cornstarch

Combine the ingredients very well with a whisk. Pour into a mason jar with holes poked into the lid. Shake the powder inside a pillowcase or under the sheets, and wake up in the morning with renewed energy after a cool, peaceful night's sleep. When storing your jar, you can place a piece of plastic wrap under the lid so that the powder won't spill out of the jar. Store in a jar with a tight-fitting lid, in a cool, dark, dry area, for up to 3 months.

UTOPIA AIR

This is the recipe I run in my diffuser if I am nervous or anxious about the upcoming day. This can make me smile no matter what mood I'm in. If my husband is feeling grumpy, I run this little gem of a combination and he is better able to handle my over-the-top personality. The curative properties in these essential oils include antidepressant, invigorating, stimulant, and sudorific.

YIELD: 1 APPLICATION

2 drops peppermint oil
2 drops neroli oil
2 drops jasmine oil

2 drops rose oil
Water

Most diffusers come with directions for using essential oils. Add the manufacturer's recommended amount of water and the oils to the diffuser and run your delightful diffuser several times a day to receive the desired effect.

CHILL OUT BATH SALTS

Use these salts in your bath when you just want to forget about the problems that are filling you with dread. This blend will transport you to another place where you can calm yourself and get ready to face the world with an open mind and heart. The properties in these oils include antidepressant, sedative, and nervine composites.

YIELD: 5 TO 6 APPLICATIONS

5 drops petitgrain oil
5 drops orange oil
5 drops neroli oil
2 tablespoons carrier oil
3 cups salts (pink Himalayan salt, sea salt, or Epsom salts)
1 tablespoon milk (optional for adults, recommended for children)

Add the essential oils and carrier oil to the salt. Stir until the oil and salt mixture is well blended. Put into a jar with lid. Let sit for 24 hours and stir again. Do not make the bathwater too hot, as the oils will dissipate. Do not add the salts when the water is running, but add ½ cup of the bath salt mixture and the milk to the water as you get into the tub. Oftentimes people add 1 tablespoon milk to the water; this will cause the essential oil to blend into the water and not float on top. Store the remainder in a jar with a tight-fitting lid, in a cool, dark area, for up to 3 months.

ARTHRITIS

There are over a hundred different types of arthritis. Arthritis is caused when the joints become inflamed. Many people contribute extreme arthritis pain to the weather, heredity, and lifestyle. Essential oils and the plants from which they are derived have long been used to reduce inflammation and relieve the pain of arthritis.

Essential Oils: sweet birch, myrrh, lemon, marjoram, peppermint, German chamomile, oregano, vetiver, eucalyptus, frankincense, geranium, ginger, lime, sandalwood, sage, pine, black pepper, camphor, tea tree (melaleuca), cedarwood, clove, thyme, and benzoin

ACHE AWAY BATH

Those aches and pains will dissipate after you linger in these essential oils' healing powers. This blend is well known for providing comfort and healing to those with arthritis. With its anti-inflammatory, sudorific, and analgesic properties, this recipe will bring relief quickly.

YIELD: 1 APPLICATION

3 drops German chamomile oil
4 drops tea tree (melaleuca) oil
3 drops myrrh oil
4 drops lime oil
1 tablespoon carrier oil
1 tablespoon milk (optional for adults, recommended for children)

As the bathwater is running, pour the ingredients into the bath. Make sure that the water is not too hot, as it will cause the essential oils to dissipate. Oftentimes people add 1 tablespoon milk to the water; this will cause the essential oil to blend into the water and not float on top. Soak in the water as long as you are comfortable.

RUB IT GOOD

This rub is good enough to use every day in your quest to end the pain that plagues you. Make pain a distant memory with this essential oil blend best known for its analgesic and anti-inflammatory properties.

YIELD: 2 TO 6 APPLICATIONS

5 drops lavender oil
3 drops lemon oil
1 drop frankincense oil
2 tablespoon carrier oil

In a small container, drip the essential oils. Pour in the carrier oil and swirl to mix the oils. Rub the affected area lightly with your fingertips or a cloth dipped in the mixture. You can also pour it into a roll-on bottle and roll onto the desired area. Be sure not to get any into the eyes or sensitive areas. Store unused portion in a jar with a tight-fitting lid, in a cool, dark area, for up to 3 months.

PRESS IT IN!

Just apply this compress to your aching bones while you relax or watch TV. The healing power of the analgesic, anti-inflammatory, and anesthetic properties of these essential oils will draw out the pain and leave you feeling refreshed and energized.

YIELD: 1 TO 2 APPLICATIONS

2 drops peppermint oil
2 drops vetiver oil
1 drop ginger oil

1 drop oregano oil
1 tablespoon carrier oil

Use gauze, linen, or any comfortable, clean cloth. Drip the ingredients onto the cloth and place over the affected area. Leave for 5 to 10 minutes. Repeat as often as needed. Remove immediately should any burning or itching occur. Store the remainder in a jar with a tight-fitting lid, in a cool, dark area, for up to 1 month.

ARTHRITIC BATH SALTS

These healing salts will become a staple when you see their effects on your pain. The bath, the salts, and the essential oils with their analgesic and anti-inflammatory properties all work together to get you back to the perfection that you know is you! When my arthritis has me feeling like an old lady, this is the bath I use to restore my vigor and vitality and end my pain.

YIELD: 5 TO 6 APPLICATIONS

5 drops ginger oil
5 drops tea tree (melaleuca) oil
5 drops sage oil
2 tablespoons carrier oil
3 cups salts (pink Himalayan salt, sea salt, Epsom salts)
1 tablespoon milk (optional for adults, recommended for children)

Add the essential oils and carrier oil to the salt. Stir until the oil and salt mixture is well blended. Put into a jar with a lid. Let sit for 24 hours and stir again. Do not make the bathwater too hot, as the oils will dissipate. Do not add the salts when the water is running, but add ½ cup of the bath salt mixture and the milk to the water as you get into the tub. Oftentimes people add 1 tablespoon milk to the water; this will cause the essential oil to blend into the water and not float on top. Store the remainder in a jar with a tight-fitting lid, in a cool, dark area, for up to 3 months.

ATHLETE'S FOOT

A fungal attack on the feet. There are many creams and lotions on the market today dealing with chronic athlete's foot. The plants and herbs from which we get our essential oils have been used for thousands of years to end fungal infections and protect the skin.

Essential Oils: tea tree (melaleuca), peppermint, patchouli, eucalyptus, lemon, cypress, lavender, thyme, myrrh, sandalwood, clove, geranium, lemongrass, and benzoin

FUNGAL FIGHTING POWDER

My husband just sprinkles this powder into his socks before he puts them on. The essential oils are healing and preventative in the fight against fungus. He used to get athlete's foot quite often, but has not had an outbreak in a long, long time since using this powder. These essential oils contain antibacterial, antibiotic, antifungal, and anti-infectious properties to fight fungus.

Yield: 10 to 20 applications

7 drops tea tree (melaleuca) oil
4 drops geranium oil
4 drops sage oil
¼ cup cornstarch

Mix the ingredients together in a plastic bag or a jar with holes punched in the lid. When storing your jar, you can place a piece of plastic wrap under the lid so that the powder won't spill out of the jar. Apply to the feet three times daily, especially after showering. Store in a jar with a tight-fitting lid, in a cool, dark, dry area, for up to 3 months.

KUNG FU FUNGAL KNOCKOUT

This wash is perfect to use before bedtime so that the essential oils can work their magic all night long. This recipe is full of antifungal, antibiotic, and anti-infectious properties to give you the relief and healing you require.

YIELD: 1 APPLICATION

10 drops tea tree (melaleuca) oil
4 drops geranium oil
2 drops thyme oil
1 ounce apple cider vinegar

Mix the ingredients in a bowl and stir. Wash the affected area with the mixture as often as needed. Use throughout the day and discard any remainder at the end of the day.

THE GOOD RUB

Apply this 3 or 4 times throughout the day to end the fungal nightmare and get your skin back to its soft self. These healing essential oils are perfect little fungus fighters with their antifungal properties. Be careful, though: oil is slippery!

YIELD: 2 TO 6 APPLICATIONS

2 drops lavender oil
2 drops tea tree (melaleuca) oil
2 drops thyme oil
1 ounce carrier oil

Combine the ingredients in a bottle. Shake before using. Apply to the feet as often as needed. Store unused portion in a jar with a tight-fitting lid, in a cool, dark area, for up to 3 months.

BACK PAIN

There are many potential causes of back pain, including wearing improper shoes, the wrong diet, disease, and physical damage in any area of the spine or neck. It is recommended that you see a physician or a chiropractor to diagnose and treat chronic back pain. However, a diagnosis doesn't guarantee that you'll discover the cause. Plants and herbs have been used for thousands of years to bring relief to those suffering from back pain.

Essential Oils: cajeput, birch, thyme, black pepper, peppermint, marjoram, rosemary, frankincense, helichrysum, lemon, sandalwood, white fir, wintergreen, basil, eucalyptus, lavender, oregano, myrrh, lime, arnica, and chamomile

LAY IT ON ME!

This recipe is a favorite in our family when it comes to lower back pain. It eases the pain and comforts the soul. When back pain hits, it can be devastating. I have only been bedridden twice in my life, and one of those times was from excruciating pain in my lower back. It is very frustrating to lose all of you to pure pain. My daughter used several of these oils on my back and I slowly was able to eradicate the back pain altogether due to the analgesic, antispasmodic, anti-inflammatory, and tonic properties.

YIELD: 1 APPLICATION

3 drops myrrh oil
2 drops helichrysum oil
2 drops thyme oil
1 ounce carrier oil

Use gauze, linen, or any comfortable, clean cloth. Place the ingredients on the cloth and place over the affected area. Leave on for as long as it is comfortable. Repeat as often as needed.

RUB THAT PAIN AWAY

Of course when you have back pain, a nice rub is the way to go. When you include these essential oils in the mix, it doubles the pleasure by providing you with healing benefits and as an added boost you can enjoy the pleasing aromas, physical contact, and the massage you receive. This blend contains healing properties from analgesic, anesthetic, antispasmodic, sedative, and anti-inflammatory agents.

YIELD: 4 TO 10 APPLICATIONS

4 drops sandalwood oil
4 drops arnica oil
2 drops peppermint oil
1 drop rosemary oil

1 drop marjoram oil
2 ounces carrier oil

In a small container, drip the essential oils. Pour in the carrier oil and swirl to mix the oils. Rub the painful area lightly to ensure that the essential oils are distributed over the skin. You can also pour it into a roll-on bottle and roll onto the desired area. Be sure not to get any into the eyes or sensitive areas. Store the remainder in a jar with a tight-fitting lid, in a cool, dark area, for up to 3 months.

GETTING OUT THE KINKS BATH SALTS

Bath salts are the bomb! You can make up a batch so that they will be ready for you when you are having a very bad back day. These salts will be ready to bring you relief and comfort when you feel you can't go one more minute without some real reprieve from the constant pain. The soothing elements of this blend include antidepressant, anti-inflammatory, sedative, antispasmodic, and cooling properties.

YIELD: 5 TO 6 APPLICATIONS

5 drops chamomile oil
5 drops rosemary oil
5 drops lime oil
2 tablespoons carrier oil

3 cups salts (pink Himalayan salt, sea salt, Epsom salts)

1 tablespoon milk (optional for adults, recommended for children)

Add the essential oils and carrier oil to the salt. Stir until the oil and salt mixture is well blended. Put into a jar with a lid. Let sit for 24 hours and stir again. Do not make the bathwater too hot, as the oils will dissipate. Do not add the salts when the water is running, but add ½ cup of the bath salt mixture and the milk to the water as you get into the tub. Oftentimes people add 1 tablespoon milk to the water; this will cause the essential oil to blend into the water and not float on top. Store the remainder in a jar with a tight-fitting lid, in a cool, dark area, for up to 3 months.

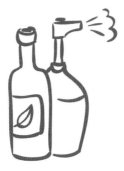

BAD BREATH
(Halitosis)

This can be caused by anything from eating garlic to gum disease. If you think your bad breath stems from a medical condition, please see a physician or dentist for relief. Many people with halitosis have gone on to a much sweeter-smelling lifestyle as a result of essential oils.

Essential Oils Used: lavender, clove, fennel, cardamom, myrrh, bergamot, and peppermint

GARGLE AND SPIT

This remedy is strong to last long! Lavender contains antifungal, anti-inflammatory, antiseptic, antiviral, and bactericidal properties. As for the brandy, alcohol is included in many mouthwashes because it kills germs and prevents infections that often lead to halitosis. Just make sure not to swallow it!

YIELD: 1 TO 2 APPLICATIONS

4 drops lavender oil
1 teaspoon brandy
¾ cup water

Be sure that the oils you use are specifically

labeled that they can be taken internally. Mix the essential oils with the water and brandy. Swish in your mouth or gargle for 30 seconds, then spit it out. Store unused portion in a jar with a tight-fitting lid, in a cool, dark area or in the refrigerator, for 1 day.

NO MORE STINKY BREATH!

Myrrh has the ability to not only get rid of your bad breath, but to protect your mouth for hours from those germs responsible for halitosis. The good-breath-promoting agents in myrrh contain antibacterial, antifungal, antimicrobial, antiseptic, and astringent properties.

YIELD: 1 TO 2 APPLICATIONS

1 drop myrrh oil
½ cup water

Be sure that the oils you use are specifically labeled that they can be taken internally. Combine the ingredients in a glass and swish in your mouth or gargle for 30 seconds, then spit it out. Store unused portion in a jar with a tight-fitting lid, in a cool, dark area or the refrigerator, for 1 day.

RINSE IT CLEAN

Everybody who's ever popped a mint knows that peppermint oil can make your breath smell wonderful. Try this little essential oil remedy and you will be hooked! Peppermint oil contains antifungal, anti-inflammatory, and antiseptic properties.

YIELD: 1 TO 2 APPLICATIONS

2 drops peppermint oil
½ cup water

Be sure that the oil you use is specifically labeled that it can be taken internally. Combine the ingredients in a glass and swish in your mouth or gargle for 30 seconds, then spit it out. Store unused portion in a jar with a tight-fitting lid, in a cool, dark area or the refrigerator, for 1 day.

BED WETTING
(Enuresis)

There are myriad reasons why a person who has the ability to walk to the bathroom might one day wake up in a puddle. It is best to consult a physician to find out what the underlying issues are. Oftentimes enuresis is thought to be brought on by stress, insomnia, and worry. Many young men experience enuresis, but usually outgrow it. Never apply essential oils to the genital area.

Essential Oils: cypress, cilantro, lavender, and chamomile

WAKE ME UP IN TIME! FOOT RUB

The feet are one of the best places to absorb essential oils into every cell in the body. This foot rub helps the body to relax so you can sleep when you are supposed to sleep, and wake when you are supposed to awaken. The therapeutic properties in this recipe are antidepressant, nervine, and sedative.

YIELD: 1 APPLICATION

2 drops chamomile oil

Apply 1 drop oil to the sole of each foot and re-apply as often as needed.

BODY RELAXATION RUB

Calm your stress and relax your worries with this gentle rubdown. This recipe contains the all-natural healing compounds of antidepressant, sedative, and nervine elements.

YIELD: 2 TO 6 APPLICATIONS

3 drops cilantro oil
3 drops lavender oil
3 drops cypress oil
1 ounce carrier oil

In a small container, drip the essential oils. Pour in the carrier oil and swirl to mix the oils. Rub the neck and back area lightly to ensure that the essential oils are distributed evenly over the skin. You can also pour it into a roll-on bottle and roll onto the desired area. Be sure not to get any into the eyes or sensitive areas. Store un-used portion in a jar with a tight-fitting lid, in a cool, dark area, for up to 3 months.

MASSAGE ME INTO THE DREAM WORLD

It is thought that stress and worry lead to enuresis. Ensure that you are going to sleep peacefully with this light massage of essential oils. These oils contain sedative, nervine, antidepressant, and restorative properties.

YIELD: 2 TO 6 APPLICATIONS

3 drops chamomile oil
3 drops cypress oil
2 drops lavender oil
1 ounce carrier oil

Place the essential oils in a small container. Pour in the carrier oil and swirl to mix the ingredients. Use your fingertips or a cloth dipped in the mixture to lightly massage the abdomen, neck, and back. Keep the essential oil mixture away from open wounds or sensitive areas. This can be repeated as needed. Store unused portion in a jar with a tight-fitting lid, in a cool, dark area, for up to 3 months.

BIPOLAR DISORDER

Some believe that this condition is hereditary, as usually more than one person in a family suffers from bipolar disorder, a mental illness characterized by a period of mania followed by a period of depression. Many drugs are available today to assist people with managing their mood swings, and various therapies have proven to be beneficial. Essential oils, herbs, and home remedies have been successfully used by thousands of people to level out their moods and to keep them from going to extremes. Therapy is also very helpful so that a person does not sink into despair from depression. It is imperative that people suffering from bipolar disorder seek treatment and consult with their medical team about using essential oils and herbs in conjunction with their medications.

Essential Oils: melissa, frankincense, rose, clary sage, vetiver, basil, and lavender

BIPOLAR POWDER

With this powder under your sheets, it's hard to lie in bed and dwell on the negative aspects of life. Bring your racing mind under control and begin to dream again with these essential oils that contain all-natural antidepressant, sedative, and nervine components. This powder has been proven to work by many of the bipolar friends and family members in my life and they often call in a panic to say that they need more!

YIELD: 10 TO 20 APPLICATIONS

3 drops melissa oil
3 drops clary sage oil
3 drops vetiver oil
¼ cup cornstarch

Combine the ingredients very well with a whisk. Pour into a mason jar with holes poked into the lid. Shake the powder inside a pillowcase or under the sheets, and wake up in the morning with renewed energy after a cool, peaceful night's sleep. When storing your jar, you can place a piece of plastic wrap under the lid so that the powder won't spill out of the jar. Store in a jar with a tight-fitting lid, in a cool, dark, dry area, for up to 3 months.

VANNOY'S AIR

This diffuser recipe keeps a positive, insightful blend of aromas in the air. These essential oils were derived from plants used for thousands of years to bring harmony to the mind. The therapeutic properties contained in this oil are aphrodisiac, euphoric, and hypertensive. When we have big family gatherings, this is the blend I often use to uplift spirits and keep everyone from killing each other.

YIELD: 1 APPLICATION

3 drops lavender oil
3 drops clary sage oil
Water

Most diffusers come with directions for using essential oils. Add the manufacturer's recommended amount of water and the oils to the diffuser and run your delightful diffuser several times a day to receive the desired effect.

RUB OUT MANIA

Before you get to that manic stage of spending all the money, moving all the furniture, and quitting your job, try this rub to bring those impulsive ideas back down to Earth. This recipe has essential oils that contain antidepressant, sedative, and tranquilizing properties.

YIELD: 1 APPLICATION

1 drop vetiver oil
1 drop frankincense oil
1 teaspoon carrier oil

In a small container, drip the essential oils. Pour in the carrier oil and swirl to mix the oils. With your fingertips or a soft cloth, rub the area around the neck and temples lightly to ensure that the essential oils are distributed evenly. You can also pour it into a roll-on bottle and roll onto the desired area. Be sure not to get any into the eyes or sensitive areas. If any of the mixture remains, store in a container with a tight-fitting lid in the refrigerator for up to 3 days.

BLEEDING

If you're bleeding from a small cut or wound, applying pressure to the site can often stop it. If bleeding is severe or an artery or vein has been punctured, this is a medical emergency and you must seek medical intervention. The following recipes are for a small cut or wound, for which essential oils can assist in the healing process.

Essential Oils: tea tree (melaleuca), geranium, chamomile, and lemon

STOP THE BLOOD PRESS

Apply this press to a small cut or wound to stop

the bleeding immediately and help keep the wound from getting infected. Some of the therapeutic oils in this recipe contain hemostatic and styptic agents to stop the flow of blood.

YIELD: 1 APPLICATION

1 drop geranium oil
1 drop lemon oil
1 drop chamomile oil
1 drop tea tree (melaleuca) oil
1 teaspoon carrier oil

Use gauze, linen, or any comfortable, clean cloth. Drip the ingredients onto the cloth and place over the affected area while applying light pressure. If any of the mixture remains, store in a container with a tight-fitting lid in the refrigerator for up to 3 days.

BLOATING

This uncomfortable feeling can be caused by countless issues such as overeating, menses, alcohol, salt, and illness. Numerous essential oils are derived from plants that are known diuretics and will help detox your body by eliminating waste.

Essential Oils: juniper, fennel, black pepper, sandalwood, rosemary, geranium, frankincense, patchouli, citrus, grapefruit, cedarwood, cypress, chamomile, citrus, and benzoin

WAIST WASTE

These oils can help you lose some of the water weight and ease any bloating with their diuretic properties.

YIELD: 1 TO 2 APPLICATIONS

3 drops juniper oil
2 drops chamomile oil
2 drops sandalwood oil
1 drop black pepper oil
1 tablespoon carrier oil

In a small container, drip the essential oils. Pour in the carrier oil and swirl to mix the oils. Rub the lower abdomen area lightly with your fingertips or a soft cloth to ensure that the essential oils are distributed over the skin. You can also pour into a roll-on bottle and roll onto the desired area. Be sure not to get any into the eyes or sensitive areas. Store the remainder in a jar with a tight-fitting lid, in a cool, dark area, for up to 1 month.

P'D OFF

This recipe will have you running to the bathroom, and your abdomen will soon be shrinking. Just make sure you don't stray too far from a restroom—these diuretic essential oils work well to end that bloat and bring back that flat tummy.

YIELD: 1 TO 2 APPLICATIONS

1 drop fennel oil
2 drops black pepper oil
2 drops lavender oil
2 drops cypress oil
1 tablespoon carrier oil

In a small container, drip the essential oils. Pour in the carrier oil and swirl to mix the oils. Rub the lower abdomen area lightly with your fingertips or a soft cloth dipped into the mixture to ensure that the essential oils are distributed over the skin. You can also pour into a roll-on bottle and roll onto the desired area. Be sure not to get any into the eyes or sensitive areas. Store the remainder in a jar with a tight-fitting lid, in a cool, dark area, for up to 1 month.

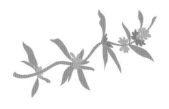

BOILS

An angry, red, swollen area of skin full of pus from infection and dead tissue. If it's in a very tender location, or badly infected, it may need to be lanced by a medical professional. Essential oils can help to alleviate the pain that is associated with boils and bring them to a head so that the pressure can be relieved.

Essential Oils: tea tree (melaleuca), frankincense, lemon, bergamot, clove, thyme, lavender, rosemary, juniper, helichrysum, geranium, and oregano

BOIL BANDAGE

These essential oils can help bring a painful boil to a head with their analgesic, anti-infectious, antibacterial, and drawing compounds. Boils are painful, ugly, and a nuisance. Butt boils are the worst! This salve on a bandage will heal it up in no time.

YIELD: 1 APPLICATION

2 drops tea tree (melaleuca) oil
1 drop clove oil
1 drop oregano oil
½ teaspoon carrier oil

Mix the ingredients well. Apply a few drops of the ingredients to a bandage or a piece of gauze with a cotton swab and secure to the site. Do not place directly on genitals or other sensitive areas. Leave on for several hours or overnight. If any of the mixture remains, store in a container with a tight-fitting lid in the refrigerator for up to 3 days.

BOIL SOAKER COMPRESS

The essential oils in this recipe have properties that are pain-relieving, analgesic, anti-inflammatory, and antibacterial, and can help bring a boil to a head and protect you from infection.

YIELD: 1 TO 2 APPLICATIONS

2 drops tea tree (melaleuca) oil
2 drops juniper oil
2 drops thyme oil
1 drop lemon oil
1 tablespoon carrier oil

Mix the ingredients in a small bowl or cup. Use gauze, linen, or any comfortable, clean cloth. Place the ingredients on the cloth and place over the affected area for 15–30 minutes, or as long as is comfortable for you. You may secure cloth or gauze to area if desired with tape or bandage. Store the remainder in a jar with a tight-fitting lid, in a cool, dark area, for up to 1 month.

A WATCHED BOIL NEVER BOILS

This is an excellent recipe to carry with you, so you can apply it to your boil often during the day. These essential oils have analgesic, astringent, antiseptic, and antibruising properties.

YIELD: 4 TO 10 APPLICATIONS

3 drops frankincense oil
3 drops helichrysum oil
2 drops lavender oil
1 ounce carrier oil

In a small container, drip the essential oils. Pour in the carrier oil and swirl to mix the oils. Dip your fingertips or a cloth into the mixture and rub the affected area lightly to ensure that the essential oils are distributed evenly over the skin. You can also pour it into a roll-on bottle and roll onto the desired area. Be sure not to get any into the eyes or sensitive areas. Store the remainder in a jar with a tight-fitting lid, in a cool, dark area, for up to 3 months.

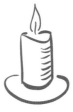

BRONCHITIS

An inflammation of the mucous membranes of the lungs. Many people get repeated bouts of bronchitis throughout their lives. Medical professionals can prescribe medicine to ensure it does not turn into pneumonia in severe cases. Essential oils can alleviate some of the congestion and breathing issues associated with bronchitis.

Essential Oils: clove, frankincense, benzoin, basil, lavender, tea tree (melaleuca), pine, eucalyptus, oregano, peppermint, thyme, marjoram, cypress, lemon, angelica, camphor, cedarwood, cajeput, niaouli, hyssop, helichrysum, myrrh, melissa, lime, and manuka

BETTER BREATHING AIR

This recipe will keep everyone in the home breathing well. Eucalyptus oil has been used for many centuries to relieve pulmonary issues. This blend contains anti-inflammatory, antiviral, antispasmodic, expectorant, and mucolytic agents to break up congestion, relieve pain, and get you back on your feet quickly.

YIELD: 1 APPLICATION

3 drops eucalyptus oil
3 drops rosemary oil

Water

Most diffusers come with directions for using essential oils. Add the manufacturer's recommended amount of water and the oils to the diffuser and run your delightful diffuser several times a day to receive the desired effect.

BREATHING BETTER RUB

This recipe is perfect for an overnight rub. These essential oils have been used for years for those suffering from coughing, mucous excess, and bronchitis. Cough-relieving and healing agents in this recipe include anti-infectious, antiphlogistic, and decongestant properties.

YIELD: 2 TO 6 APPLICATIONS

2 drops clove oil
2 drops frankincense oil
1 drop peppermint oil
1 ounce carrier oil

In a small container, drip the essential oils. Pour in the carrier oil and swirl to mix the oils. Rub the chest, back, or back of neck area lightly to ensure that the essential oils are distributed over the skin. You can also pour it into a roll-on bottle and roll onto the desired area. Be sure not to get any into the eyes or sensitive areas. Store unused portion in a jar with a tight-fitting lid, in a cool, dark area, for up to 3 months.

PRANAYAMA BATH

Pranayama is the Indian word for "breath," so this recipe is all about getting you back to breathing your best. This is full of lung-clearing essential oils that will help relieve a stuffy head and chest quickly with ingredients such as antispasmodic, antiviral, decongestant, and expectorant compounds, to name a few. So take a leisurely bath and get yourself well today.

YIELD: 1 APPLICATION

3 drops eucalyptus oil
2 drops pine oil
1 drop lemon oil
1 drop myrrh oil
1 drop manuka oil
1 tablespoon carrier oil
1 tablespoon milk (optional for adults,
    recommended for children)

As the bathwater is running, pour the ingredients into the bath. Make sure that the water is not so hot as to cause the essential oils to dissipate. Oftentimes people add 1 tablespoon milk to the water; this will cause the essential oil to blend into the water and not float on top. Soak in the water as long as you are comfortable.

BURNS

Mild burns can be treated with essential oils for immediate relief. More severe burns should be seen and treated by a medical professional. For on-the-spot relief, lavender is often the essential oil of choice for minor surface burns, as it can be applied neat.

Essential Oils: chamomile, rose, lavender, helichrysum, tea tree (melaleuca), frankincense, geranium, neroli, thyme, peppermint, white fir, rosemary, sage, niaouli, manuka, clove, and eucalyptus

BOO-BOO MILD BURN BANDAGE

This recipe is great for children; they won't even know you put a drop of these mild oils on their bandage, yet the healing effects for mild burns are astounding and sometimes seem even miraculous. I always keep a vial of lavender oil in the kitchen for those inevitable steam burns. One drop later and I can't even find where I burned myself. The healing properties in some of these oils are analgesic, anti-inflammatory, antiseptic, and bactericidal agents.

YIELD: 1 APPLICATION

2 drops lavender oil

1 drop thyme oil

1 drop sage oil

½ teaspoon carrier oil

Mix the ingredients well. Apply a few drops of the mixture to a bandage or a piece of gauze with an eye dropper and secure the bandage to the site. Leave on for several hours or overnight. Reapply as needed. If any of the mixture remains, store in a container with a tight-fitting lid in the refrigerator for up to 3 days. If applying to bandage or skin, use a cotton swab or cotton ball to apply to avoid getting fingertips in oil.

OUCH RELIEF

These are the all-time go-to oils for burns in our home. They can be placed on the skin neat to bring instant relief. The cicatrisant, antibiotic, and analgesic properties of these oils are well known for their burn-healing magic.

YIELD: 1 APPLICATION

1 drop lavender oil, or 1 drop frankincense oil

Apply with a cotton swab to the sore and leave it on the area. A few essential oils can be placed directly on the skin without adding carrier oil to them. Be sure that you are using a safe essential oil before placing it on the body, as essential oils can be very powerful. Be sure the burn is not an open wound. Essential oils applied neat are for very mild wounds only.

WASH THAT BURN

This is great for a burn that also needs washing to remove dirt and particles. Ensure that it is a mild burn and that the skin is not broken. If the skin is broken, you may need to seek medical attention. A few of the healing agents in these oils are disinfectant, bactericidal, cicatrisant, and analgesic properties.

YIELD: 1 APPLICATION

5 drops lavender oil

3 drops frankincense oil

4 ounces water

Combine ingredients in a bowl. With a soft washcloth, apply the mixture to the affected area and let air dry. Never apply to an open wound or near sensitive body parts. Dispose of any remainder. Reapply daily.

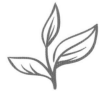

CARPAL TUNNEL SYNDROME

When the median nerve in the carpal tunnel is compressed, this can cause intense pain, swelling, and a number of other complaints. It is believed that repetitive movements, such as working at a computer or on an assembly line, are the culprits behind this painful condition. Treatment involves resting the hand, placing the hand in a splint, and putting ice packs on the wrist. Surgery often helps with reducing the effects of this syndrome. Essential oils can alleviate pain and reduce swelling at the site of nerve damage.

Essential Oils: frankincense, cypress, helichrysum, oregano, chamomile, clove, basil, birch, lemongrass, sandalwood, peppermint, and marjoram

DAMN! THAT HURTS WRIST RUB

Carpal tunnel is extremely painful. When you don't want to take medication, this is a good rub that helps make that pain more bearable. I had an extreme case of carpal tunnel for about six months, and I applied this every day for relief and comfort to my wrist. The essential oils in this recipe contain pain-fighting agents with analgesic, anti-inflammatory, antibruising, and sedative properties.

YIELD: 2 TO 6 APPLICATIONS

3 drops chamomile oil
3 drops marjoram oil
3 drops helichrysum oil
1 ounce carrier oil

In a small container, drip the essential oils. Pour in the carrier oil and swirl to mix the oils. Rub the area lightly to ensure that the essential oils are distributed evenly over the skin. You can also pour it into a roll-on bottle and roll onto the desired area. Be sure not to get any into the eyes or sensitive areas. Store unused portion in a jar with a tight-fitting lid, in a cool, dark area, for up to 3 months.

REAL GOOD RELIEF RUB

Rub this on when you are having pain and can't take medications. These essential oils have been crucial for years for relieving pain with their analgesic, bactericidal, antivenous, anti-infectious, and antibiotic properties.

YIELD: 2 TO 6 APPLICATIONS

4 drops lemongrass oil
4 drops lavender oil

1 ounce carrier oil

In a small container, drip the essential oils. Pour in the carrier oil and swirl to mix the oils. Rub the area lightly to ensure that the essential oils are distributed over the skin. You can also pour it into a roll-on bottle and roll onto the desired area. Be sure not to get any into the eyes or sensitive areas. Store unused portion in a jar with a tight-fitting lid, in a cool, dark area, for up to 3 months.

WRIST WRAP

This is an excellent wrap recipe that you can leave on overnight for all-night-long relief and have a better day tomorrow. I used this at night to prevent myself from waking up in screaming pain. It worked very well for me. The properties at work to bring you pain relief in this recipe are analgesic, antibacterial, anti-inflammatory, antioxidant, and antiseptic components.

YIELD: 2 TO 6 APPLICATIONS

3 drops cypress oil
2 drops sandalwood oil
2 drops peppermint oil
1 ounce carrier oil

Apply a tablespoon of the ingredients to a long piece of muslin or cotton. Wrap the treated material around the wrist. Leave for at least 15 minutes. Store unused portion in a jar with a tight-fitting lid, in a cool, dark area, for up to 3 months.

CATARRH

This is a thick collection of mucus often caused by colds, flu, allergies, or other ailments. Catarrh often causes discomfort and sleeplessness for patients. If it's not corrected it can lead to complications such as pneumonia or bronchitis, so it's best to see a medical professional for diagnosis. Essential oils can help with the fatigue, coughing, and other physical discomforts brought on by catarrh.

Essential Oils: peppermint, niaouli, myrrh, eucalyptus, thyme, ginger, tea tree (melaleuca), manuka, cajeput, lime, lemon, cedarwood, lavender, jasmine, pine, sandalwood, and rosemary

MAKE ME BETTER MASSAGE

This recipe is great to bring relief to the lungs. These essential oils have long been known to bring much-needed clearing and dispelling of mucus. The agents at work in this recipe include analgesic, antibacterial, decongestant, and expectorant properties.

YIELD: 2 TO 6 APPLICATIONS

3 drops tea tree (melaleuca) oil
3 drops eucalyptus oil
3 drops rosemary oil
1 ounce carrier oil

Place the essential oils in a small container. Pour in the carrier oil and swirl to mix the ingredients. Use your fingertips or a cloth to apply and lightly massage the chest, back, or the area desired. Keep the mixture away from open wounds or sensitive areas. This can be repeated as needed. Store unused portion in a jar with a tight-fitting lid, in a cool, dark area, for up to 3 months.

LET'S CLEAR THE AIR

This is a diffuser recipe that will have the whole household breathing easier. These essential oils have been used for years, and the plants they're derived from have been used to clear lungs and sinuses for centuries. When my husband is congested, he will tell me to "go plug in that machine." I will put these oils in the diffuser and he can then breathe so much better. A few of the agents at work here in these oils have antispasmodic, decongestant, expectorant, and analgesic properties.

YIELD: 1 APPLICATION

2 drops eucalyptus oil
2 drops cajeput essential oil
2 drops pine oil
Water

Most diffusers come with directions for using essential oils. Add the manufacturer's recommended amount of water and the oils to the diffuser and run your delightful diffuser several times a day to receive the desired effect.

COUGH-RELIEVING BATH SALTS

Bath salts can be considered a personal indulgence, but they have powerful healing properties when these oils are added. This blend contains analgesic, febrifuge, decongestant, and bactericidal properties.

YIELD: 5 TO 6 APPLICATIONS

5 drops pine oil
5 drops eucalyptus oil
5 drops niaouli oil
2 tablespoons carrier oil
3 cups salts (pink Himalayan salt, sea salt, or
   Epsom salts)
1 tablespoon milk (optional for adults,
   recommended for children)

Add the essential oils and carrier oil to the salt.

Stir until the oil and salt mixture is well blended. Put in jar with lid. Let sit for 24 hours and stir again. Do not make the bathwater too hot, as the oils will dissipate. Do not add the salts when the water is running, but add ½ cup of the bath salt mixture and the milk to the water as you get into the tub. Oftentimes people add 1 tablespoon milk to the water; this will cause the essential oil to blend into the water and not float on top. Store the remainder in a cool, dark area, in a jar with a tight-fitting lid, for up to 3 months.

CELLULITE

A condition that affects mostly women, cellulite has an array of causes, including genetics, exercise and diet, hormones stress, and hormones. Essential oils have shown varying degrees of success in treating cellulite.

Essential Oils: grapefruit, geranium, cypress, helichrysum, thyme, lavender, myrrh, lemon, frankincense, wild birch, sandalwood, and juniper

SMOOTH THIS UGLY OUT

The plants from which these essential oils are derived have been used forever to help women get rid of bumpy cellulite skin and smooth it out for that youthful look. The skin-smoothing agents here include circulatory, revitalizing, cicatrisant, and tonic properties.

YIELD: 4 TO 10 APPLICATIONS

3 drops helichrysum oil
2 drops lavender oil
2 drops myrrh oil
1 ounce carrier oil

Place the essential oils in a small container. Pour in the carrier oil and swirl to mix the ingredients. Use your fingertips or a cloth to lightly massage the cellulite area. Keep the mixture away from open wounds or sensitive areas. This can be repeated as needed. Store the remainder in a jar with a tight-fitting lid, in a cool, dark area, for up to 3 months.

RUB IT LIKE A GENIE

This recipe can smooth out textured skin when used repeatedly. The therapeutic properties include cytophylactic, restorative, and vasoconstrictor agents.

YIELD: 4 TO 10 APPLICATIONS

3 drops cypress oil
2 drops grapefruit oil

2 drops geranium oil
2 ounces carrier oil

In a small container, drip the essential oils. Pour in the carrier oil and swirl to mix the oils. Using your fingertips or a cloth, rub the area lightly to ensure that the essential oils are distributed over the skin. You can also pour it into a roll-on bottle and roll onto the desired area. Be sure not to get any into the eyes or sensitive areas. Store the remainder in a jar with a tight-fitting lid, in a cool, dark area, for up to 3 months.

BATHE THESE LUMPS AWAY

This bath recipe has rich, cellulite-fighting essential oils with astringent, tonic, and stimulant properties, as well as circulatory, diuretic, and depurative agents.

YIELD: 1 APPLICATION

3 drops grapefruit oil
2 drops juniper oil
1 drop lemon oil
1 drop myrrh oil
1 tablespoon carrier oil
1 tablespoon milk (optional for adults,
 recommended for children)

As the bathwater is running, pour the ingredients into the bath. Make sure that the water is not so hot as to cause the essential oils to dissipate. Oftentimes people add 1 tablespoon milk to the water; this will cause the essential oil to blend into the water and not float on top. Soak in the water as long as you are comfortable.

CHAPPED LIPS

The rough, dry, scaly feeling of the lips can be caused by a variety of factors such as illness, dehydration, and weather. There are many essential oils that can help alleviate chapped lips.

Essential Oils: lavender, frankincense, aloe vera, sandalwood, chamomile, tea tree (melaleuca), rose, neroli, and geranium

KISS ME OIL

Who can resist these soft lips after applying the essential oils in this recipe? Soothing and softening agents include emollient, anti-inflammatory, cytophylactic, and cicatrisant properties.

YIELD: 20 TO 60 APPLICATIONS

1 ounce aloe vera oil
2 drops geranium oil

2 drops rose oil
1 drop chamomile oil

Combine all the ingredients in a small jar or tin. When your lips feel chapped or dry, apply to the lips liberally with your fingertips. Repeat as often as necessary. Store unused portion in a jar with a tight-fitting lid, in a cool, dark area, for up to 3 months.

JUICY ROLLER

Help smooth out those fine lines and make your lips plump and smooth. The essential oils in this recipe soften the skin while healing with cicatrisant, antiseptic, vulnerary, and antiviral therapeutic properties.

YIELD: 10 TO 20 APPLICATIONS

4 drops frankincense oil
4 drops lavender oil
1 drop rose oil
1 teaspoon carrier oil

Place the ingredients in a roller bottle. Roll onto the lips as often as desired.

Store the remainder in a jar with a tight-fitting lid, in a cool, dark area, for up to 1 month.

CIRCULATION (POOR)

This condition is achieved by various factors. Standing too long, standing on concrete, illness, and age are among the myriad of reasons a person might have poor circulation. Some essential oils may increase blood circulation that can help restore circulation, movement, and energy to your limbs.

Essential Oils: black pepper, ginger, cypress, lemongrass, neroli, eucalyptus, lemon, geranium, coriander, citrus, thyme, bay laurel, ylang-ylang, rose, lime, benzoin, cinnamon, marjoram, basil, sandalwood, myrrh, peppermint, and frankincense

SUPERFAST HEATING MASSAGE

The essential oils in this recipe can get the blood moving and help end the pain. But never rub too hard, as blood clots can be moved and cause adverse reactions, stroke, or death. The blood-circulating properties in this blend include antibruising, anti-inflammatory, anticoagulant, and cicatrisant agents.

2 drops cypress oil

2 drops lemon oil

2 drops frankincense oil

1 drop helichrysum oil

1 ounce carrier oil

Place the essential oils in a small container. Pour in the carrier oil and swirl to mix the ingredients. Use to lightly massage the target area to heat the area and get the blood circulating. Keep the mixture away from open wounds or sensitive areas. This can be repeated as needed. Store unused portion in a jar with a tight-fitting lid, in a cool, dark area, for up to 3 months.

SOOTHING MASSAGE OIL

Massage this oil in very lightly and enjoy the healing benefits of these essential oils with their anti-inflammatory, circulation-boosting agents.

2 drops cypress oil

2 drops neroli oil

2 drops lemon oil

2 drops eucalyptus oil

1 drop frankincense oil

1 ounce carrier oil

Place the essential oils in a small container. Pour in the carrier oil and swirl to mix the in-

gredients. Use your fingertips or a small cloth to lightly massage the target area. Keep the mixture away from open wounds or sensitive areas. This can be repeated as needed. Store unused portion in a jar with a tight-fitting lid, in a cool, dark area, for up to 3 months.

BLOOD CIRCULATION BATH

This bath uses essential oils that reportedly help with circulation, and it feels good too! I have poor circulation in my feet, and during the winter they are bitterly cold. Taking this bath gets my blood pumping, and my feet stay warm for the rest of the day. The circulating properties in this recipe include tonic, depurative, and cicatrisant components.

2 drops orange oil

2 drops lemongrass oil

2 drops neroli oil

1 drop black pepper oil

3 drops rose oil

1 tablespoon carrier oil

1 tablespoon milk (optional for adults, recommended for children)

While the bathwater is running, pour the ingredients into the bath. Make sure that the water is not so hot as to cause the essential oils to dissi-

pate. Oftentimes people add 1 tablespoon milk to the water; this will cause the essential oil to blend into the water and not float on top. Soak in the water as long as you are comfortable.

COLDS

Fever, chills, coughing, and a runny nose are just some of the symptoms of the common cold, which is caused by a virus that typically attacks the throat, nose, chest, and head areas, making you feel tired, run down, and moody. Essential oils can help prevent a cold, and also alleviate some of the symptoms if you've already got one.

Essential Oils: cajeput, eucalyptus, pine, frankincense, lime, lemon, lavender, peppermint, basil, cinnamon, rosemary, neroli, manuka, juniper, helichrysum, camphor, bergamot, clove, niaouli, thyme, tea tree (melaleuca), oregano, cypress, and cassia

STAY-AWAY AIR FRESHENER

Keep the germs away with this delightful blend that not only smells good, but also works double-time to keep you and your family safe and healthy. A few of the protecting properties in this blend include antifungal, anti-infectious, antiviral, and antiseptic agents.

Yield: 1 application

3 drops lemon oil
2 drops eucalyptus oil
3 drops frankincense oil
4 drops peppermint oil
Water

Most diffusers come with directions for using essential oils. Add the manufacturer's recommended amount of water and the oils to the diffuser and run your delightful diffuser several times a day to receive the desired effect.

NIGHTY-NIGHT SLEEP TIGHT RUB

This recipe has oils in it that not only help you sleep well, but also fight germs while you sleep to protect you against cold and flu germs. Some of the sleep-inducing and protectant therapeutic properties that I crave when needing a good night's sleep include anti-inflammatory, bactericidal, sedative, and antibiotic compounds.

Yield: 2 to 6 applications

3 drops eucalyptus oil
2 drops lavender oil
2 drops oregano oil

1 drop niaouli oil
1 ounce carrier oil

In a small container, drip the essential oils. Pour in the carrier oil and swirl to mix the oils. Rub the chest and neck area lightly with your fingertips or a small cloth to ensure that the oils are distributed over the skin. You can also pour into a roll-on bottle and rolled onto the desired area. Be sure not to get any into the eyes or sensitive areas. Store unused portion in a jar with a tight-fitting lid, in a cool, dark area, for up to 3 months.

GET ME THROUGH THE DAY PROTECTION BATH

This recipe can help you to breathe better while protecting you at the same time. Airways will open and breathing becomes easier with the decongestant, antimicrobial, expectorant, and mucolytic properties contained in this recipe.

YIELD: 1 APPLICATION

6 drops lavender oil
5 drops eucalyptus oil
3 drops pine oil
1 tablespoon carrier oil
1 tablespoon milk (optional for adults,
*   recommended for children)*

While the bathwater is running, pour the ingredients into the bath. Make sure that the water is not so hot as to cause the essential oils to dissipate. Oftentimes people add 1 tablespoon milk to the water; this will cause the essential oil to blend into the water and not float on top. Soak in the water as long as you are comfortable.

COLD SORES

Also known as herpes simplex or fever blisters, these viral sores typically affect the same people over and over. Although there's no known cure for cold sores, essential oils can help prevent an outbreak.

Essential Oils: tea tree (melaleuca), clove, peppermint, melissa, sandalwood, myrrh, eucalyptus, bergamot, lemongrass, niaouli, chamomile, calendula, geranium, lavender, frankincense, lemon, thyme, lime, and ravensara

SPOT ON

These essential oils can be applied neat and will bring instant relief while healing your cold sore. The therapeutic properties that impart quick healing include antibacterial, antibiotic, and antifungal functions.

YIELD: 1 APPLICATION

*1 drop frankincense oil, or 1 drop tea tree
(melaleuca) oil, or 1 drop lavender oil*

Apply with a cotton swab to the sore and leave it on the area. A few essential oils can be placed directly on the skin (neat) without adding carrier oil to them. Be sure that you are using a safe and pure essential oil before placing on the body, as essential oils can be very powerful.

RUB IT AWAY

This roll-on can be carried in your purse and applied liberally throughout the day. The essential oils have long been reputed to keep the herpes virus at bay and to heal your cold sore once it's emerged with their antifungal, antibiotic, and anti-inflammatory healing agents. You will soon find yourself smiling again without any pain!

YIELD: 10 TO 20 APPLICATIONS

2 drops eucalyptus oil
2 drops tea tree (melaleuca) oil
1 drop clove oil
1 teaspoon carrier oil

In a small container, drip the essential oils. Pour in the carrier oil and swirl to mix the oils. Rub the area lightly with a cotton swab dipped in the mixture to ensure that the oils are distributed over the outbreak. You can also pour it into a roll-on bottle and roll onto the desired area. Be sure not to get any into the eyes or sensitive areas.

Store the remainder in a jar with a tight-fitting lid, in a cool, dark area, for up to 1 month.

CLEANSING BATH

Because essential oils are absorbed through the skin and carried to every cell of your body, ridding your system of toxins, viruses, and bacteria, this bath recipe can help clear up those stubborn sores. Some of the healing agents included in this recipe are anti-inflammatory, antimicrobial, depurative, expectorant, and immune-stimulating properties.

YIELD: 1 APPLICATION

3 drops rose oil
2 drops tea tree (melaleuca) oil
2 drops lavender oil
2 drops niaouli oil
1 drop lemongrass oil
1 tablespoon carrier oil
*1 tablespoon milk (optional for adults,
recommended for children)*

As the bathwater is running, pour the ingredients into the bath. Make sure that the water is not so hot as to cause the essential oils to dissipate. Oftentimes people add 1 tablespoon milk to the water; this will cause the essential oil to blend into the water and not float on top . Soak in the water as long as you are comfortable.

CONCENTRATION

The inability to focus for extended periods of time is termed a lack of concentration. There are mitigating circumstances that could cause a person to be unable to concentrate: exhaustion, anxiety, even hunger. Essential oils can increase not only your focus and concentration, but your memory as well.

Essential Oils: bergamot, vetiver, basil, cedarwood, peppermint, cardamom, wild birch, rosemary, and rose

CONCENTRATION POWDER

Focus on your sleep and get your mind right for the day ahead using this recipe. The plants that these essential oils were derived from have been reputed for centuries to help people achieve focus. Some of the sleep-inducing properties in this recipe are antidepressant, nervine, and tranquilizing agents.

YIELD: 10 TO 20 APPLICATIONS

3 drops vetiver oil
3 drops cardamom oil
3 drops rose oil
¼ cup cornstarch

Combine the ingredients very well with a whisk. Pour into a mason jar with holes poked into the lid. Shake the powder inside a pillowcase or under the sheets, and wake up in the morning with renewed energy after a cool, peaceful night's sleep. When storing your jar, you can place a piece of plastic wrap under the lid so that the powder won't spill out of the jar. Store in a jar with a tight-fitting lid, in a cool, dark, dry area for up to 3 months.

FOCUS INHALATION

Do you have a big test or interview coming up and need to focus? Inhaling the aroma of these essential oils will keep your mind on track. Since menopause, I use these oils often to help me focus throughout the day. They have long been known to contain memory-enhancing properties. Some of the agents at work in this recipe are restorative, tonic, and stimulant therapeutic properties.

YIELD: 1 APPLICATION

1 drop peppermint oil, or 1 drop lemon oil, or 1 drop rosemary oil

Place the drop of essential oil onto a handkerchief, tissue, in the palm of your hand, or into an essential oil inhaler. Cup to your nose and inhale the aroma. Repeat several times daily or as needed.

CONCENTRATION SPRITZ

Keep this spray in your purse for when you are faced with a task that you need to concentrate on. You can spray this on your clothes or in the air and get ready to have pinpoint focus. The oils work together, with their stimulating and tonic properties, to enhance your memory and focus.

YIELD: 50 TO 100 SPRAYS PER 4-OUNCE BOTTLE

2 drops cardamom oil
2 drops rose oil
2 drops vetiver oil
2 drops peppermint oil
4 ounces water

Combine the essential oils and the water in a 4-ounce spray bottle. Lightly spritz onto the desired area. Allow to air dry. The essential oils will be absorbed by the skin on contact and also be breathed into the respiratory chambers. Store in the spray bottle in a cool, dark area, for up to 3 months.

CONGESTION

This condition is caused when the mucous membranes of the nose, throat, or chest become inflamed. There are many reasons for congestion, including colds, tonsillitis, adenoid inflammation, and a variety of illnesses. Essential oils can lessen the side effects of congestion and have been reported to reduce congestion. If congestion interferes with breathing or becomes chronic, seek medical assistance.

Essential Oils: ginger, thieves', eucalyptus, peppermint, cedarwood, tea tree (melaleuca), bergamot, benzoin, thyme, clove, birch, cypress, marjoram, sandalwood, allspice, black pepper, frankincense, basil, and pine

RELIEVING SMELLING SALTS

Carry a little vial of this mixture in your purse and you will be ready at a moment's notice to relieve that congestion and clear your head. The plants these essential oils are derived from have been used for centuries to alleviate the congestion that accompanies colds and flu. The therapeutic properties at work in this blend are expectorant, anti-inflammatory, and decongestant.

YIELD: ½ TEASPOON

5 drops eucalyptus oil
½ teaspoon sea salt or kosher salt

Combine the essential oil with the salt. Place in a small vial and inhale the scent as needed. Replace with new salts and essential oils monthly. Store in a dry, dark area.

VAPOR RUB

This is a great little rub to use at bedtime; you will sleep without having your breathing constricted. These essential oils will open the airways and bring your breathing under control with their decongestant, antispasmodic, antimicrobial, and analgesic therapeutic properties.

YIELD: 4 TO 10 APPLICATIONS

6 drops eucalyptus oil
2 drops peppermint oil
2 drops thyme oil
2 drops lemon oil
1 drop black pepper oil
2 ounces carrier oil

In a small container, drip the essential oils. Pour in the carrier oil and swirl to mix the oils. Rub the chest area lightly with your fingertips or a small, clean cloth to ensure that the oils are distributed over the skin. You can also pour it into a roll-on bottle and roll onto the desired area. Be sure not to get any into the eyes or

sensitive areas. Store the remainder in a jar with a tight-fitting lid, in a cool, dark area, for up to 3 months.

FOG-LIFTING AIR

This diffuser recipe not only helps me when I am feeling congested, but also when I'm suffering from other minor ailments such as nausea or fatigue. I just feel generally crappy when I am congested and I need to have healing elements all around me. The therapeutic properties of the oils in this recipe include antispasmodic, bactericidal, sudorific, and tonic agents.

YIELD: 1 APPLICATION

4 drops ginger oil
3 drops cypress oil
Water

Most diffusers come with directions for using essential oils. Add the manufacturer's recommended amount of water and the oils to the diffuser and run your delightful diffuser several times a day to receive the desired effect.

CONSTIPATION

The inability to have a normal bowel movement. There are so many reasons that a person may suffer from constipation that they can't all be listed here. Diet, lack of exercise, medications, nerves—the list is endless. The essential oils in this recipe, when rubbed on the abdomen, have been reputed to help persons with elimination and get back to feeling worth a poop!

Essential Oils: marjoram, fennel, yarrow, black pepper, tarragon, rosemary, lemon, orange, cinnamon, thyme, sandalwood, ginger, lemon, peppermint, and cassia

SOFTEN IT UP

The abdomen rub is one of the oldest known remedies in human history. Try this recipe to help loosen up the bowels with its antiemetic, antispasmodic, detoxifying, and digestive properties.

YIELD: 2 TO 6 APPLICATIONS

3 drops fennel oil
2 drops yarrow oil
2 drops thyme oil
1 drop black pepper oil
1 ounce carrier oil

Place the essential oils in a small container. Pour in the carrier oil and swirl to mix the oils. Use your fingertips or a soft cloth to lightly massage the abdomen area. Keep the mixture away from open wounds or sensitive areas. This can be repeated as needed. Store unused portion in a jar with a tight-fitting lid, in a cool, dark area, for up to 3 months.

LOOSEN IT UP BATH

This recipe and the heat from the bath work in conjunction to bring you the relief you seek. The therapeutic properties in this blend include analgesic, antispasmodic, carminative, laxative, stomachic, and bactericidal elements.

YIELD: 1 APPLICATION

3 drops rosemary oil
3 drops orange oil
2 drops marjoram oil
1 drop peppermint oil
1 drop pine oil
1 tablespoon carrier oil
1 tablespoon milk (optional for adults,
    recommended for children)

While the water is running, pour the ingredients into the bath. Make sure that the water is not so hot as to cause the essential oils to dissipate. Oftentimes people add 1 tablespoon milk to the water; this will cause the essential oil to blend into the water and not float on top of the water. Soak in the water as long as you are comfortable.

FULL OF IT RUB

When you're full of it and don't want it, this rub will help get rid of it. The therapeutic properties in this blend contain antispasmodic, analgesic, stomachic, and laxative properties.

Yield: 4 to 10 applications

5 drops rosemary oil
3 drops marjoram oil
3 drops peppermint oil
1 drop sandalwood oil
2 ounces carrier oil

In a small container, drip the essential oils. Pour in the carrier oil and swirl to mix the oils. Rub the abdomen area lightly with your fingertips or a soft cloth to ensure that the oils are distributed over the skin. You can pour it into a roll-on bottle and roll onto the desired area. Be sure not to get any into the eyes or sensitive areas. Store the remainder in a jar with a tight-fitting lid, in a cool, dark area, for up to 3 months.

COUGH

The cough reflex helps rid the body of an unwanted particle in the lungs. Illness, allergies, asthma, smoking, and a host of other factors can introduce the coughing reflex in people. Essential oils have been used for centuries to suppress a cough, or at least make it more productive. But if your cough is chronic or severe, seek medical attention.

Essential Oils: peppermint, eucalyptus, thyme, tea tree (melaleuca), melissa, pine, lemon, oregano, hyssop, niaouli, benzoin, cypress, white fir, lavender, clove, and anise

QUIET-TIME SYRUP

This is the recipe I used on my daughters when they were young. When a trip to the doctor wasn't in our budget, we had to make do with what we had. This is an economical recipe that tastes good and brings quick results. It's a wonderful syrup for bedtime, as it has essential oils that will keep you from coughing all night long. The therapeutic elements of this recipe include analgesic, antibacterial, and anti-inflammatory components along with decongestant properties.

Yield: 1 application

1 drop cinnamon oil
2 drops lemon oil
3 tablespoons honey
1 cup warm water

Be sure that the oils you use are clinical grade and specifically labeled that they can be taken internally. Mix the ingredients in a cup and sip slowly. Store the remainder in the refrigerator and drink within 24 hours.

THROAT RELIEVER

Too much coughing can irritate the lining of the throat. These essential oils have healing properties that can relieve that sore throat and bring about a quick recovery. This recipe includes antibacterial and antimicrobial components.

YIELD: 1 TO 2 APPLICATIONS

1 drop cinnamon oil
1 drop lemon oil
2 ounces water

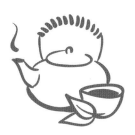

Be sure that the oils you use are clinical grade and specifically labeled that they can be taken internally. Mix the oils and water. Swish in the mouth and gargle, then spit it out. Store the remainder in a jar with a tight-fitting lid, in the refrigerator, for up to 24 hours.

I JUST WANT TO BREATHE RUB

This rub is great for bedtime and can help you sleep through the night without waking up every 5 minutes to cough. The properties that are included in this blend are analgesic, antibacterial, anti-inflammatory, antimicrobial, antiseptic, and decongestant.

YIELD: 2 TO 6 APPLICATIONS

3 drops eucalyptus oil
3 drops peppermint oil
2 drops cypress oil
2 tablespoons carrier oil

In a small container, drip the essential oils. Pour in the carrier oil and swirl to mix the oils. Rub the chest or back area lightly with your fingertips or a soft cloth to ensure that the essential oils are distributed over the skin. You can pour it into a roll-on bottle and roll onto the desired area. Be sure not to get any into the eyes or sensitive areas. Store unused portion in a jar with a tight-fitting lid, in a cool, dark area, for up to 3 months.

CUTS

Essential oils are used to speed the healing process of minor cuts and fight against infection. If cuts are deep or severe, seek medical attention, as stitches may be needed. While you should never put essential oils directly into a deep cut or gaping wound that goes through several layers of skin, minor cuts and wounds can benefit from essential oil applications.

Essential Oils: helichrysum, benzoin, frankincense, myrrh, tea tree (melaleuca), lavender, eucalyptus, rose, chamomile, lemon, and geranium

GOD'S BANDAGE

Use this age-old recipe to heal a minor cut. These essential oils are known worldwide for the speedy healing effects of their cicatrisant, anti-inflammatory, antiseptic, and analgesic components.

YIELD: 1 APPLICATION

1 drop lavender oil
1 drop frankincense oil
1 drop myrrh oil

Place the oils on and around the cut with a cotton swab and cover with gauze and tape, or place the oils on the bandage with a swab.

Watch closely for infection and change the bandage periodically.

BOO-BOO SPRAY

This recipe doesn't sting, and children love it. I keep this spray handy all summer when my grandchildren like to run outside, invariably coming into the house with wounds, bruises, and laughter. Keep it handy to use daily as needed. The essential oils in this recipe are used worldwide for minor cuts and wounds. The antiseptic, antibacterial, and hepatic properties in this recipe bring quick healing.

YIELD: 50 TO 100 SPRAYS PER 4-OUNCE BOTTLE

8 drops lavender oil
3 drops tea tree (melaleuca) oil
2 drops eucalyptus oil
2 drops chamomile oil
1 drop rose oil
4 ounces water

Combine the ingredients in a 4-ounce spray bottle and lightly spray the affected area. Allow to air dry. Repeat as needed. Store in the spray bottle in a cool, dark area, for up to 3 months.

HEALING SALVE

A great healing salve for minor cuts, wounds, and burns. These easily recognizable essential oils are quick and effective at healing and protecting from inflammation and infection with their antibiotic, antibacterial, anti-infectious, and antimicrobial properties. This salve is like a miracle to us, and is also used throughout my family for sprains, bruises, sore muscles, burns, and rashes.

YIELD: 10 TO 20 APPLICATIONS

¼ to ½ ounce beeswax

1 tablespoon olive oil (or other suitable carrier oil)

5 drops tea tree (melaleuca) oil

4 drops helichrysum oil

4 drops myrrh oil

4 drops frankincense oil

2 drops vitamin E oil

Heat the beeswax and olive oil in a microwave oven until almost melted. Stir until fully melted, let cool for a couple of minutes, and add the essential oils and vitamin E oil. Let cool to room temperature before applying to minor cuts and burns. Refrigerate in a small container with a tight-fitting lid when not in use.

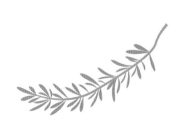

DEPRESSION

There can be many reasons for a person to suffer from depression. Oftentimes a person feels lethargic or sad and can't find a valid reason for feeling this way. The plants, trees, and shrubs from which we get our essential oils have been used for thousands of years as a way of dispelling the feelings of doom and gloom often associated with depression. Occasional bouts of depression are a factor of human existence and have been experienced by everyone. But when that depression is severe or lingers for an extended amount of time, affecting our family and our careers, we should seek professional intervention. A college professor told me many years ago that maybe people suffering from depression are the ones who are right, and everyone else is just looking at the world through rose-colored glasses. Regardless if it is normal or not, depression should be taken seriously.

Essential Oils: vetiver, neroli, petitgrain, sandalwood, ylang-ylang, bergamot, orange, clary sage, cypress, cedarwood, geranium, rose, lemon, marjoram, frankincense, lime, melissa, tea tree (melaleuca), patchouli, wild orange, rosemary, basil, cinnamon, and all spice oils

DEPRESSION POWDER

Depression and bipolar disorder run in my family. This is a timeless recipe we use to give the suffering family member rest and happy thoughts. Put this powder between the sheets so your loved one can have a great night's sleep without worrisome thoughts thanks to the restorative, antidepressant, and tranquilizing properties of this blend.

Yield: 10 to 20 applications

3 drops wild orange oil
3 drops rosemary oil
3 drops vetiver oil
¼ cup cornstarch

Combine the ingredients very well with a whisk. Pour into a mason jar with holes poked into the lid. Shake the powder inside a pillowcase or under the sheets, and wake up in the morning with renewed energy after a cool, peaceful night's sleep. When storing your jar, you can place a piece of plastic wrap under the lid so that the powder won't spill out of the jar. Store in a jar with a tight-fitting lid, in a cool, dark, dry area, for up to 3 months.

RUB IT AND MAKE IT BETTER

This rub can bring instant relief, and you can apply it to yourself or your family members.

When you are down in the dumps, lift your soul and your spirit with these mood-lightening essential oils that contain nervine, antidepressant, euphoric, and sedative elements. This blend can make me feel better even if I do have something concrete to be depressed about.

Yield: 4 to 10 applications

3 drops neroli oil
2 drops patchouli oil
2 drops ylang-ylang oil
2 drops tea tree (melaleuca) oil
2 drops cypress oil
1 drop basil oil
2 ounces carrier oil

In a small container, drip the essential oils. Pour in the carrier oil and swirl to mix the oils. Rub the neck and temples lightly with your fingertips or a soft cloth to ensure that the essential oils are distributed over the skin. You can also pour it into a roll-on bottle and roll onto the desired area. Be sure not to get any into the eyes or sensitive areas. Store the remainder in a jar with a tight-fitting lid, in a cool, dark area, for up to 3 months.

HAPPY, HAPPY, HAPPY SPRAY

Carry this spray with you to use on yourself, in your car, or at your office. These oils can lift the spirits and soothe the soul with their aphrodisiac, restorative, stimulating, and tonic boosting properties. So put down the wine, pick up the spray, and have yourself a great day—with no hangover!

YIELD: 50 TO 100 SPRAYS PER 4-OUNCE BOTTLE

2 drops rose oil
2 drops sandalwood oil
2 drops frankincense oil
2 drops bergamot oil
1 drop rosemary oil
4 ounces water

Combine the ingredients in a 4-ounce spray bottle and shake well before using. Spray into rooms, cars, on linen, or on yourself. This is a great uplifting aroma that will bring a smile to anyone's face. Store in the spray bottle in a cool, dark area for up to 3 months.

DERMATITIS

This is another name for eczema, an itching, cracking, weeping area of skin. Eczema is very hard to heal in most cases, and it usually takes a very long time to understand its root cause. I suffered for decades before discovering that wheat and sugar were the causes of my particular case. When I have a flare-up of eczema, essential oils are brought into play to calm my skin.

Essential Oils: thyme, comfrey, calendula, geranium, tea tree (melaleuca), rosemary, peppermint, lavender, birch, helichrysum, Roman chamomile, sage, chamomile, frankincense, lemon, myrrh, oregano, clary sage, patchouli, palmarosa, juniper, and cedarwood

ITCH-RELIEVING COMPRESS

When the rash starts itching, make it disappear by using these essential oils to soothe and soften and make skin feel wonderful. The therapeutic properties at work here are antibiotic, anti-inflammatory, antiseptic, hydration, and detoxifying agents. Get rid of that itchy alligator skin and bring back that sexy, smooth skin.

YIELD: 2 TO 6 APPLICATIONS

3 drops lavender oil
3 drops tea tree (melaleuca) oil
2 drops palmarosa oil
1 ounce carrier oil

Use gauze, linen, or any comfortable, clean cloth. Place the mixed ingredients on the cloth and place over the affected area. Leave on as long as your are comfortable, 15 to 30 minutes. Store unused portion in a jar with a tight-fitting lid, in a cool, dark area, for up to 3 months.

DRY SKIN BATH

Take a bath and moisturize your skin at the same time with these juicy essential oils! The all-natural healing benefits of this recipe include anti-inflammatory, astringent, circulatory, vulnerary, and cicatrisant properties. Luxuriate in this bath: you deserve it!

YIELD: 1 APPLICATION

3 drops myrrh oil
3 drops helichrysum oil
3 drops tea tree (melaleuca) oil
1 tablespoon carrier oil
1 tablespoon milk (optional for adults, recommended for children)

While the bathwater is running, pour the ingredients into the bath. Make sure that the water is not so hot as to cause the essential oils to dissipate. Oftentimes people add 1 tablespoon milk to the water; this will cause the essential oil to blend into the water and not float on top. Soak in the water as long as you are comfortable.

COMFORTING SALVE

This recipe is full of healing essential oils that will bring hydration back to your dry, cracked, painful skin with their cicatrisant, circulatory, immune-stimulating, and vulnerary elements. No need for expensive treatments when you have these oils in your possession!

YIELD: 2 TO 6 APPLICATIONS

½ ounce beeswax
1 tablespoon olive oil (or other suitable carrier oil)
3 drops tea tree (melaleuca) oil
3 drops lavender oil
2 drops helichrysum oil
2 drops Roman chamomile oil
2 drops vitamin E oil

Heat the beeswax and olive oil in a microwave oven until almost melted. Stir until fully melted, let cool for a couple of minutes, and add the essential oils and vitamin E oil. If too thick, add more olive oil. If too thin, add more beeswax. Let cool completely and spread on the affected area with your fingertips or a cotton swab. Store unused portion in a jar with a tight-fitting lid, in a cool, dark area, for up to 3 months.

DETOX

Whether you want to cleanse your body of a harmful substance or just feel refreshed and invigorated after a time of eating unhealthy food (or too much alcohol), detox can aid in this process. Essential oils can help in many facets of the detox process, from calming a person down to distributing essential natural components throughout the body.

Essential Oils: juniper, coriander, rose, honeysuckle, garlic, lemon, peppermint, angelica, wild birch, and fennel

DETOX POWDER

Help relieve the fidgeting and nighttime worries with this soothing, calming-for-the-soul powder. These essential oils will relax you and help you to be at your best the next day. The calming elements of these oils contain relaxant and nervine properties. I used this blend every night when I quit smoking and I ended up not killing anyone or smoking a cigarette.

YIELD: 10 TO 20 APPLICATIONS

3 drops lemon oil
3 drops fennel oil
3 drops angelica essential oil
¼ cup cornstarch

Combine all of the ingredients together in a large bowl, using a whisk. Place the mixture in a mason jar with holes poked into the lid. Shake the powder inside a pillowcase or under the sheet as needed. You can place a piece of plastic wrap under the lid to keep the powder from spilling out when not in use. Store in a jar with a tight-fitting lid, in a cool, dark, dry area, for up to 3 months.

POISON-RELEASING BATH

These essential oils are reputed to help rid your body of toxins and heal at the same time. I find that doing things that are for you and you alone can help with the detoxification process. A few of the healing benefits include antiseptic, antispasmodic, antitoxic, depurative, and detoxifying properties.

YIELD: 1 APPLICATION

4 drops lavender oil
3 drops lemon oil
2 drops juniper oil
1 cup Epsom salts
1 tablespoon carrier oil
1 tablespoon milk (optional for adults, recommended for children)

After the bathwater has run, mix the salt into the water and drip the essential oils into the bath. Make sure that the water is not so hot as to cause the essential oils to dissipate. Oftentimes people add 1 tablespoon milk to the water; this will cause the essential oil to blend into the water and not float on top. Soak in the water as long as you are comfortable.

PURE BODY DRINK

Lemon and water is considered by many to be one of the most effective combinations to rid the body of toxins with its detoxifying elements.

YIELD: 1 TO 2 APPLICATIONS

1 drop lemon oil
2 ounces water

Ensure that your essential oil is safe for consumption and internal usage and is clinical/therapeutic grade. Mix the oil with the water and drink slowly. Store unused portion in a jar with a tight-fitting lid, in a cool, dark area, or in the refrigerator for 1 day.

DIARRHEA

Often accompanied by cramping, excessive gas, bloating, and sometimes nausea, this is caused by a myriad of illnesses. Essential oils can relax the abdominal muscles when rubbed on the stomach, bringing much relief. If symptoms persist or are severe, causing dehydration, consult a physician to ensure that other factors aren't contributing to excessive bowel movements.

Essential Oils: peppermint, Roman chamomile, eucalyptus, fennel, ginger, cypress, cinnamon, black pepper, neroli, cajeput, lavender, geranium, peppermint, sandalwood, oregano, tea tree (melaleuca), clove, and thyme

SETTLE IT DOWN MASSAGE OIL

This recipe is a tummy rub intended to calm the digestive tract and put an end to that painful situation. These essential oils are known to be calming and healing due to their antispasmodic, anti-inflammatory, carminative, and digestive properties. So get off the pot and get back to having fun.

YIELD: 2 TO 6 APPLICATIONS

2 drops peppermint oil
2 drops lavender oil
2 drops chamomile oil
2 drops eucalyptus oil
2 drops geranium oil
2 tablespoons carrier oil

Place the essential oils in a small container. Pour in the carrier oil and swirl to mix the oils. Use your fingertips or a soft cloth to lightly massage the abdomen area. Keep the mixture away from open wounds or sensitive areas. This can be repeated as needed. Store unused portion in a jar with a tight-fitting lid, in a cool, dark area, for up to 3 months.

NAUSEA NO MORE DRINK

This is a time-tested recipe that will have your stomach settled in no time. Be sure to drink very slowly. This recipe is one that I also use when I eat food that doesn't agree with my digestive tract. These oils contain stomachic, carminative, and emmenagogue properties to relieve nausea and cramping.

YIELD: 1 TO 2 APPLICATIONS

2 drops peppermint oil
2 drops ginger oil
4 ounces water

Ensure that your essential oils are safe for consumption and internal use and are clinical/therapeutic grade. Mix the oils with the water and drink slowly. Store unused portion in a jar with a tight-fitting lid, in a cool, dark area or the refrigerator, for 1 day.

THE CORK

This is a pleasant, calming rub that can help to alleviate many problems associated with diarrhea. People swear by these essential oils for diarrhea and stomach issues due to their analgesic, antiemetic, and carminative agents, among others. My husband calls this recipe "The Cork" for obvious reasons.

YIELD: 2 TO 6 APPLICATIONS

3 drops Roman chamomile oil
2 drops ginger oil
2 drops neroli oil
2 drops cypress oil
2 tablespoons carrier oil

In a small container, drip the essential oils. Pour in the carrier oil and swirl to mix the oils. Rub the stomach area lightly with your fingertips or a soft cloth to ensure that the essential oils are distributed over the skin. You can also pour it into a roll-on bottle and roll onto the desired area. Be sure not to get any into the eyes or sensitive areas. Store unused portion in a jar with a tight-fitting lid, in a cool, dark area, for up to 3 months.

DIGESTION ISSUES

There are numerous reasons why a person might have digestive issues, ranging from stress to disease. It is important to discover the cause and seek medical treatment if necessary. Essential oils can assist with various stages of recovering a healthy digestion process and other issues with the digestive tract.

Essential Oils: fennel, ginger, peppermint, grapefruit, frankincense, tarragon, anise, lemongrass, dill, coriander, thyme, juniper berry, chamomile, rosemary, black pepper, and clary sage

DIGESTIVE TRACT DRINK

Is there really anything better for the tummy than peppermint oil or ginger oil? These digestive and stomachic properties work to settle, heal, and calm an upset stomach due to their anti-inflammatory and antiemetic properties. This drink is as delicious as it is healing. You have the added benefit of not consuming all of the sugar that comes in peppermint candy, but getting effective, natural peppermint instead.

Yield: 1 to 2 applications

2 drops peppermint oil
1 drop ginger oil
4 ounces water

Ensure that your essential oils are safe for consumption and internal use and are clinical/therapeutic grade. Mix the oils with the water and drink slowly. Store unused portion in a jar with a tight-fitting lid, in a cool, dark area or the refrigerator, for up to 1 day.

TUMMY RUB

These essential oils work wonders for the digestive tract with their carminative, antiemetic, and antispasmodic therapeutic properties. I have a lot of digestive problems due to celiac disease and menopause. This rub has provided me with great relief on more than one occasion.

Yield: 2 to 6 applications

2 drops peppermint oil
2 drops clary sage oil
2 drops lemongrass oil
1 ounce carrier oil

In a small container, drip the essential oils. Pour in the carrier oil and swirl to mix the oils. Rub the abdomen area lightly with your fingertips or a soft cloth to ensure that the essential oils are distributed over the skin. You can also pour it into a roll-on bottle and roll onto the desired area. Be sure not to get any into the eyes or sensitive areas. Store unused portion in a jar with a tight-fitting lid, in a cool, dark area, for up to 3 months.

FEEL BETTER BATH

Get that digestion going again by using these essential oils to bring much-needed relief while relaxing in a pleasant bath. The depurative, lipolytic, antispasmodic, and carminative properties work well together to bring relief to your digestive tract.

YIELD: 1 APPLICATION

4 drops lemongrass oil
3 drops coriander oil
2 drops chamomile oil
1 drop clary sage oil
1 tablespoon carrier oil
1 tablespoon milk (optional for adults, recommended for children)

While the bathwater is running, pour the ingredients into the bath. Make sure that the water is not so hot as to cause the essential oils to dissipate. Oftentimes people add 1 tablespoon milk to the water; this will cause the essential oil to blend into the water and not float on top. Soak in the water as long as you are comfortable.

DRY SKIN

Everyone experiences dry skin at some point in his or her life. Some people experience cracking, peeling, and chronic dry skin due to eczema, psoriasis, or a host of other conditions. Essential oils can help or even eliminate dry skin altogether when used over a period of time. They can be added to the bathwater, a compress, salves, and other vehicles to bring relief to dry skin.

Essential Oils: geranium, sandalwood, frankincense, myrrh, Roman chamomile, patchouli, oregano, tea tree (melaleuca), peppermint, cypress, lemon, ylang-ylang, and helichrysum

SCRUBBING MY SKIN MOISTLY

This recipe is full of juicy, juicy, juicy essential oils that bring moisture and relief to dry, itchy skin. The skin healing compounds in these essential oils are anti-inflammatory, antiseptic, and antifungal elements to name a few.

YIELD: 1 APPLICATION

6 drops lavender oil
2 drops frankincense oil
2 drops peppermint oil
1 drop myrrh oil
2 tablespoons oatmeal
2 tablespoons water

Combine the ingredients without mashing too much. Spread the paste, with your fingertips, onto the dry skin. Let sit for 1 minute, then gently rinse off.

MOISTURIZING LOTION

Rub this lotion on day or night. The healing, moisturizing essential oils will help you to achieve the glowing skin you've always wanted. This is an excellent recipe for aging skin with its cicatrisant, cytophylactic, and vulnerary therapeutic properties—and we all know I need all of the help I can get for my skin.

YIELD: 2 TO 6 APPLICATIONS

5 drops geranium oil
4 drops peppermint oil
3 drops tea tree (melaleuca) oil
2 drops frankincense oil
1 ounce carrier oil

In a small container, drip the essential oils. Pour in the carrier oil and swirl to mix the oils. Rub the face and neck area lightly with your fingertips or a soft cloth dipped into the mixture to ensure that the essential oils are distributed over the skin. You can also pour into a roll-on bottle and roll onto the desired area. Be sure not to get any into the eyes or sensitive areas. Store unused portion in a jar with a tight-fitting lid, in a cool, dark area, for up to 3 months.

DRY SKIN RUB

This recipe is great for skin that is starting to crack and flake. It provides healing essential oils that will repair damaged skin and leave it feeling fresh and soft. The anti-inflammatory, cicatrisant, and antifungal properties of this recipe make it ideal as a soothing rub.

YIELD: 1 APPLICATION

1 drop tea tree (melaleuca) oil
1 drop helichrysum oil
1 drop sandalwood oil
1 teaspoon carrier oil

In a small container, drip the essential oils. Pour in the carrier oil and swirl to mix the oils. Rub the dry skin area lightly with your fingertips or a soft cloth dipped into the mixture to ensure that the essential oils are distributed over the skin. You can also pour into a roll-on bottle and roll onto the desired area. Be sure not to get any into the eyes or sensitive areas. If any of the mixture remains, store in a container with a tight-fitting lid in the refrigerator for up to 3 days.

EARACHE

Pain in the ear canal is often caused by fluid buildup, swimming, colds, or a variety of other reasons. The eardrum, Eustachian tubes, and other areas of the inner ear are very sensitive. If fever or redness is present, please consult a physician. Never apply essential oils to the inside of the ear.

Essential Oils: lavender, basil, hyssop, tea tree (melaleuca), clove, oregano, eucalyptus, frankincense, peppermint, rosemary, hyssop, orange, lemon, and grapefruit

EAR RUB

This is a healing, soothing recipe to help you manage that earache pain. The essential oils used in this recipe have been used to bring relief of earaches for many years with their analgesic, antibiotic, and anti-infectious therapeutic properties.

YIELD: 1 TO 2 APPLICATIONS

3 drops lavender oil
2 drops tea tree (melaleuca) oil
1 drop clove oil
1 tablespoon carrier oil

In a small container, drip the essential oils. Pour in the carrier oil and swirl to mix the oils. Rub the outer ear area lightly with your fingertips or a soft cloth dipped into the mixture to ensure that the essential oils are distributed over the skin. Never place any essential oils directly into the ear canal. You can also pour into a roll-on bottle and roll onto the desired area. Be sure not to get any into the eyes or sensitive areas. Store the remainder in a jar with a tight-fitting lid, in a cool, dark area, for up to 1 month.

COTTON BALL SOOTHER

This is an old recipe that brings instant relief and comfort to a person suffering from a painful earache. Basil oil contains analgesic, antibacterial, antibiotic, anti-inflammatory, and antiseptic properties, to name a few.

YIELD: 1 APPLICATION

2 drops basil oil

Place the drops of essential oil on a cotton ball, being careful to not get the liquid on your fingers. Place the cotton ball in the ear, but do not press or push into the ear canal, and let sit for 15 to 30 minutes. Repeat throughout the day as needed.

EAR MASSAGE

These essential oils are known to stop pain and bring relief to your aching ear and jaw. The properties responsible for relieving pain in these oils are analgesic, anti-inflammatory, and antiseptic agents.

YIELD: 1 APPLICATION

1 drop grapefruit oil
1 drop clove oil
1 drop lavender oil
1 teaspoon grapeseed oil

In a small container, drip the essential oils. Pour in the grapeseed oil and swirl to mix the oils. Rub the outer ear and jaw area lightly with your fingertips or a soft cloth dipped into the mixture to ensure that the essential oils are distributed over the skin. Never place any essential oils directly into the ear canal. You can also pour into a roll-on bottle and roll onto the desired area. Be sure not to get any into the eyes or sensitive areas. If any of the mixture remains, store in a container with a tight-fitting lid in the refrigerator for up to 3 days.

ECZEMA

A skin condition that is lifelong and has no known cure, eczema is often caused by food allergies—mainly wheat, eggs, sugar, or dairy—or stress. Essential oils can be most helpful in curbing outbreaks and preventing new ones. Under a doctor's guidance, a person should consider changing their diet, eliminating suspected foods and waiting to introduce them many months later after no sign of eczema is present. My entire family has celiac disease and all suffer from skin conditions, especially eczema. These recipes have helped many in my family get through those bad breakouts.

Essential Oils: helichrysum, thyme, geranium, lavender, chamomile, rosemary, neem, frankincense, comfrey, calendula, birch, tea tree (melaleuca), melissa, grapefruit, sage, lemon, myrrh, and bergamot

BATHING THE BUMPS OUT SALTS

Your skin will glow and you will feel silky smooth all over after taking this bath. Stop that itching, scaly eczema in its tracks with this blend. The essential oils in this recipe have long been known to bring comfort and healing to those suffering from eczema because of the anti-inflammatory, cicatrisant, and antiseptic properties.

YIELD: 5 TO 6 APPLICATIONS

5 drops grapefruit oil
5 drops bergamot oil
5 drops geranium oil
5 drops calendula oil
1 tablespoon carrier oil
3 cups salts (pink Himalayan salt, sea salt, or
    Epsom salts)
1 tablespoon milk (optional for adults,
    recommended for children)

Add the essential oils and carrier oil to the salt. Stir until the oil and salt mixture is well blended. Put into a jar with a lid. Let sit for 24 hours and stir again. Do not make the bathwater too hot, as the oils will dissipate. Do not add the salts when the water is running, but add ½ cup of the bath salt mixture and the milk to the water as you get into the tub. Oftentimes people add 1 tablespoon milk to the water; this will cause the essential oil to blend into the water and not float on top. Store the remainder in a jar with a tight-fitting lid, in a cool, dark area, for up to 3 months.

KICK-ASS SUPER SALVE

We love this salve in our family. It has brought so much relief to our skin many times over. Give it a try and you won't ever want to be without it. These essential oils are believed to help with many skin diseases and you can find them in tons of skin-soothing recipes. The therapeutic properties contained in these oils, to name a few, are antiallergenic, anti-infectious, anti-inflammatory, antimicrobial, and cicatrisant.

YIELD: 2 TO 6 APPLICATIONS

4 drops tea tree (melaleuca) oil
4 drops chamomile oil
2 drops lavender oil
1 drop helichrysum oil
1 ounce carrier oil

In a small container, drip the essential oils. Pour in the carrier oil and swirl to mix the oils. Rub the affected area lightly with your fingertips or a soft cloth dipped into the mixture to ensure that the essential oils are distributed over the skin. You can also pour into a roll-on bottle and roll onto the desired area. Be sure not to get any into the eyes or sensitive areas. Store unused portion in a jar with a tight-fitting lid, in a cool, dark area, for up to 3 months.

MY SPECIAL OINTMENT

Powerful healing essential oils bring a halt to painful eczema. I have used this recipe for years on my feet and have had great results due to the antiallergenic, anti-inflammatory, and cicatrisant components in this blend. This is good to keep on hand, in your purse or your car.

YIELD: 4 TO 10 APPLICATIONS

5 drops thyme oil
5 drops rosemary oil
5 drops melaleuca (tea tree) oil
5 drops helichrysum oil
2 ounces carrier oil

In a small container, drip the essential oils. Pour in the carrier oil and swirl to mix the oils. Rub the eczema area lightly with your fingertips or a soft cloth dipped into the mixture to ensure that the essential oils are distributed over the skin. You can also pour into a roll-on bottle and roll onto the desired area. Be sure not to get any into the eyes or sensitive areas. Store the remainder in a jar with a tight-fitting lid, in a cool, dark area, for up to 3 months.

ENERGY (LOW)

Energy is something that usually comes from within, but sometimes people suffering from depression, fatigue, heartbreak, grief, or illness find that they have a lack of energy and do not have the desire to do anything. Essential oils can help you regain the will to join the outside world and forge ahead.

Essential Oils: peppermint, lemon, eucalyptus, grapefruit, frankincense, bergamot, pine, clove, basil, black pepper, lemongrass, fir, cypress, cinnamon, patchouli, and sage

ENERGIZING BATH SALTS

Best morning bath ever! You will be able to think quicker and more clearly with these oils in your system. Your multitasking skills will de-velop exponentially and you can get more done than you dreamed of. Go ahead . . . try it! You will be up and running in no time as the tonic, antidepressant, energy-producing, and restor-ative properties of these essential oils work on your system.

YIELD: 5 TO 6 APPLICATIONS

7 drops frankincense oil
7 drops cypress oil
7 drops bergamot oil
2 tablespoons carrier oil
3 cups salts (pink Himalayan salt, sea salt, or
*   Epsom salts)*
1 tablespoon milk (optional for adults,
*   recommended for children)*

Add the essential oils and carrier oil to the salt. Stir until the oil and salt mixture is well blended. Put into a jar with a lid. Let sit for 24 hours and stir again. Do not make the bathwa-ter too hot, as the oils will dissipate. Do not add the salts when the water is running, but add ½ cup of the bath salt mixture and the milk to the water as you get into the tub. Oftentimes peo-ple add 1 tablespoon milk to the water; this will cause the essential oil to blend into the water and not float on top. Store the remainder in a jar with a tight-fitting lid, in a cool, dark area, for up to 3 months.

SPECIAL SPEEDY SPRAY

This is the spray I like to carry at work and it sure does make a difference when 2 or 3 o'clock rolls around. I go from rolling my eyes back into my head from midday fatigue to being Ms. Speedy due to the stimulants and invigorating properties that take effect in this blend.

YIELD: 50 TO 100 SPRAYS PER 4-OUNCE BOTTLE

6 drops peppermint oil
2 drops cinnamon oil
2 drops cypress oil
2 drops pine oil
4 ounces water

Combine the ingredients in a 4-ounce spray bottle and lightly spray the body and room area. Allow to air dry. The essential oils will be absorbed into the skin by contact or by the lungs if sprayed into the air. Store in the spray bottle, in a cool, dark area, for up to 3 months.

ENERGY PERMEATES THE AIR

This diffuse recipe has the essential oils you need to begin your day and work right through it with energy and confidence. Show everyone around you how energetic and efficient you are while running this little recipe throughout the day. The antidepressant, aphrodisiac, and tonic properties in this recipe give tons of energy and stamina to even the most sedentary of us.

YIELD: 1 APPLICATION

3 drops eucalyptus oil
3 drops patchouli oil
2 drops frankincense oil
2 drop grapefruit oil
Water

Most diffusers come with directions for using essential oils. Add the manufacturer's recommended amount of water and the oils to the diffuser and run your delightful diffuser several times a day to receive the desired effect.

EXHAUSTION

Often caused by overexertion, a person can usually overcome exhaustion by sleeping an adequate amount of time, if possible. But exhaustion can sometimes lead to hospitalization if dehydration or mental exhaustion is also present, so seek professional help if it's severe or long-lasting. Essential oils can be used to help you get back the energy and the rest you need, as you need it.

Essential Oils: rosemary, basil, wild orange, white fir, grapefruit, cassia, bergamot, peppermint, lemon, lavender, cinnamon, citrus, lime, frankincense, and eucalyptus.

GO-GO-GO RUB

This rub will lift your spirits and make you feel like you can do anything. The essential oils in this recipe are known energizers and stamina boosters. The restorative and energizing therapeutic properties in this blend will give you the energy you need to take it from a long day at work to a night on the town.

YIELD: 2 TO 6 APPLICATIONS

5 drops basil oil
1 drop cassia oil
4 drops wild orange oil
2 drops grapefruit oil
1 ounce carrier oil

In a small container, drip the essential oils. Pour in the carrier oil and swirl to mix the oils. Rub the lower abdomen area lightly with your fingertips or a soft cloth dipped into the mixture to ensure that the essential oils are distributed over the skin. You can also pour into a roll-on bottle and roll onto the desired area. Be sure not to get any into the eyes or sensitive areas. Store unused portion in a jar with a tight-fitting lid, in a cool, dark area, for up to 3 months.

ELECTRIC AIR

This diffuse is great to run during parties, events, and general activities around your home or workplace. It contains essential oils that, when they permeate the air, are reported to provide vitality to everyone around with their generally stimulating properties. You don't want a crowd of exhausted people trying to get the night over with! Turn it into a party with these awesome oils.

YIELD: 1 APPLICATION

7 drops bergamot oil
2 drops cinnamon oil
2 drops lemongrass oil
Water

Most diffusers come with directions for using essential oils. Add the manufacturer's recommended amount of water and the oils to the diffuser and run your delightful diffuser several times a day to receive the desired effect.

MORNING GET-UP BATH

It's just not fair when you wake up tired and exhausted and still have a long day to go before you are able to finally go to bed again. These essential oils help to instill energy and focus to help you forge ahead with their restorative, stimulating, and tonic properties.

YIELD: 1 APPLICATION

3 drops rosemary oil
4 drops citrus oil
2 drops white fir oil
2 drops grapefruit oil
1 tablespoon carrier oil
1 tablespoon milk (optional for adults,
  recommended for children)

While the bathwater is running, pour the ingredients into the bath. Make sure that the water is not so hot as to cause the essential oils to dissipate. Oftentimes people add 1 tablespoon milk to the water; this will cause the essential oil to blend into the water and not float on top. Soak in the water as long as you are comfortable.

EYESTRAIN

Most people are familiar with this feeling, often caused in this day and age by squinting at computers and cell phones and other eye-muscle-straining activities. Essential oils can be applied to the outer eye area to assist in relaxing the eyes and eliminate the headache and neck ache that often accompany eyestrain. Never place essential oils directly onto the eyeball or inner eyelids.

Essential Oils: lavender, chamomile, ylang-ylang, sandalwood, cypress, lemongrass, rosemary, frankincense, and helichrysum

TEA-BAGGED EYES

My sister uses this age-old recipe when her eyes give out after working at her computer all day. Chamomile is full of anti-inflammatory and muscle-relaxing properties and will give your eyes that fresh, wide-awake look.

YIELD: 1 APPLICATION

2 chamomile tea bags, soaked in warm water

Place slightly warm tea bags onto your closed eyes and allow to rest for 10 to 20 minutes.

EYE RUB

This recipe will not only help you feel alert, but will also moisturize your eye area and help you to look great as well. The properties at work here are restorative, anti-inflammatory, anti-bruising, and cicatrisant agents.

YIELD: 1 APPLICATION

1 drop helichrysum oil
1 drop frankincense oil
1 drop lavender oil
½ teaspoon carrier oil

Mix the ingredients together in a small bowl. Place the mixture on your fingertips and rub around the outer areas of the eyes, being careful to not get any on the eye itself. Do not get essential oils directly on the eyeball. Discard any remainder of the mixture.

EYE COMPRESS RELIEF

This recipe feels like a day at the spa, but has healing and strengthening essential oils in it to help you get the relief you need on your tired, overworked eyes. The anti-infectious, anti-inflammatory, and analgesic properties work together to bring healing and relief to those tired eyes.

YIELD: 1 APPLICATION

3 drops lavender oil
2 drops ylang-ylang oil
2 drops lemongrass oil
2 drops sandalwood oil
1 teaspoon carrier oil

Use gauze, linen, or any comfortable, clean cloth. Place the mixed ingredients on the cloth and place over your closed eyes. Do not get any of the mixture in the eyeballs. Relax for 10 to 20 minutes. If any of the mixture remains, store in a container with a tight-fitting lid in the refrigerator for up to 3 days.

FATIGUE

Fatigue is your body's way of telling you that you need to sleep. But sometimes it becomes so pronounced and consistent that you feel like you can't do anything but sleep! Essential oils can calm the mind and help you to sleep soundly, or they can give you enough energy to renew your spirit and help you carry on.

Essential Oils: basil, eucalyptus, lemon, grapefruit, ginger, angelica, pine, clove, black pepper, cinnamon, patchouli, lemongrass, sage, white fir, cypress, peppermint, fir, rosemary, and bergamot

ENERGY IS IN THE AIR

This diffuse recipe is great for waking everyone up and getting them moving, replacing that fatigue with an "I can do it" attitude. The stimulating and restorative properties in these oils permeate the air with electric energy to get you moving again.

YIELD: 1 APPLICATION

4 drops eucalyptus oil
3 drops bergamot oil
1 drop lemon oil
1 drop sage oil
Water

Most diffusers come with directions for using essential oils. Add the manufacturer's recommended amount of water and the oils to the diffuser and run your delightful diffuser several times a day to receive the desired effect.

WAKE ME UP INHALER

A quick, instant energizer you can use anytime, anywhere. The tonic properties of these oils give you an amazing feeling of energy and get-up-and-go, banishing fatigue instantly.

YIELD: 1 APPLICATION

1 drop basil oil, or 1 drop lemon oil, or 1 drop eucalyptus oil

Place the drop of essential oil on a handkerchief, tissue, in the palm of your hand, or into an essential oil inhaler. Cup to your nose and inhale the aroma. Repeat several times daily or as needed.

FATIGUE-FIGHTING RUB

Your skin will soak up these oils and give you the energy you need to get on with it and do it right! The essential oils in this blend work well to amp up vigor and vitality with their restorative healing properties. Fatigue: 0; energy: 1.

YIELD: 4 TO 10 APPLICATIONS

4 drops eucalyptus oil

3 drops basil oil
3 drops lemon oil
1 drop bergamot oil
1 drop cassia oil
1 drop fir oil
2 ounces carrier oil

In a small container, drip the essential oils. Pour in the carrier oil and swirl to mix the oils. Rub the temples, back of the neck, or wrist area lightly with your fingertips or a soft cloth dipped into the mixture to ensure that the essential oils are distributed over the skin. You can also pour into a roll-on bottle and roll onto the desired area. Be sure not to get any into the eyes or sensitive areas. Store the remainder in a jar with a tight-fitting lid, in a cool, dark area, for up to 3 months.

FEVER

One of the body's weapons to defend itself and try to burn out the enemy, fever can be a useful tool, but can also be potentially deadly. Fever is a symptom, usually letting us know that there is an infection somewhere inside the body, and you must investigate and get medical treatment to determine the cause. There are many options for bringing a temperature down, and essential oils have long been used to cool the body. But if the body temperature is too high or persists, you must obtain medical intervention, especially for an infant or the elderly.

Essential Oils: eucalyptus, peppermint, lime, rosemary, tea tree (melaleuca), lemon, lavender, thieves', clove, black pepper, frankincense, manuka, lavender, yarrow, basil, bergamot, cajeput, petitgrain, niaouli, camphor, cardamom, helichrysum, and lemongrass

NEAT FEVER REDUCER

A time-honored treatment that can be used to help reduce that fever and make you feel better. Peppermint oil's cooling properties have been used for generations to bring fevers down and get that patient feeling fine again.

Yield: 1 application

2 drops peppermint oil
4 drops carrier oil

Be sure that you are using a therapeutic-grade essential oil before placing it on the body, as essential oils can be very powerful. Peppermint oil can burn sensitive skin, so mixing it with a carrier oil is good practice. Always use caution when using essential oils. Rub the mixture on the neck and temples to reduce fever.

COOLING MASSAGE

The essential oils in this recipe have been known to bring down the body temperature and help cool a person off quickly due to their analgesic, anesthetic, anti-infectious, febrifuge, and anti-inflammatory properties.

Yield: 2 to 6 applications

2 drops eucalyptus oil
2 drops lavender oil
2 drops peppermint oil
1 drop lime oil
1 ounce carrier oil

In a small container, drip the essential oils. Pour in the carrier oil and swirl to mix the oils. Rub the back of the neck, chest, or temple area lightly with your fingertips or a soft cloth dipped into the mixture to ensure that the essential oils are distributed over the skin. You can also pour into a roll-on bottle and roll onto the desired area. Be sure not to get any into the eyes or sensitive areas. Store unused portion in a jar with a tight-fitting lid, in a cool, dark area, for up to 3 months.

ICEEEE DRINK

Bringing a fever down quickly is easily done with a cool glass of ice and this detoxifying and tonic-inducing essential oil–laced water. Ensure that your essential oil is safe for consumption and internal use and is clinical/therapeutic grade.

YIELD: 1 TO 2 APPLICATIONS

1 drop lemon oil
4 ounces cold water

Mix the essential oil and water and drink slowly. Store unused portion in a jar with a tight-fitting lid, in a cool, dark area or the refrigerator, for up to 1 day.

BATH COOLDOWN

These essential oils work wonders at reducing fevers, and a tepid bath will help quickly. These oils contain detoxifying, anti-inflammatory, antimicrobial, antiseptic, and bactericidal properties. When my children were younger and brought many viruses home from school, this was our go-to recipe to get that body temp back to normal.

YIELD: 1 APPLICATION

2 drops black pepper oil
6 drops eucalyptus oil
4 drops lemon oil
1 tablespoon carrier oil
1 tablespoon milk (optional for adults, recommended for children)

While the bathwater is running, pour the ingredients into the bath. Make sure that the water is not so hot as to cause the essential oils to dissipate. Oftentimes people add 1 tablespoon milk to the water; this will cause the essential oil to blend into the water and not float on top. Soak in the water as long as you are comfortable.

FLU

Influenza is a contagious disease that causes coughing, sore throat, fever, headache, chills, and a variety of other symptoms. The main worry when having the flu is that it will lead to more serious illnesses such as pneumonia and bronchitis. Essential oils can alleviate many symptoms and bring relief. Seek medical intervention if the flu lasts longer than a few days or if symptoms are severe.

Essential Oils: eucalyptus, frankincense, lemon, lavender, thieves', peppermint, oregano, marjoram, rosemary, cypress, cinnamon, cassia, basil, hyssop, chamomile, bergamot, thyme, clove, pine, and melaleuca (tea tree)

FLU-FIGHTING POWDER

During flu season, we keep this powder between our sheets and mattress to protect us from flu germs while we sleep. It will also help someone who has had the flu recover while protecting him or her from reinfection. These protective essential oils all have properties reputed to fight flu germs and bring about restored health such as antibacterial, antibiotic, anti-infectious, and anti-inflammatory agents.

YIELD: 10 TO 20 APPLICATIONS

3 drops oregano oil
3 drops thieves' oil
3 drops tea tree (melaleuca) oil
¼ cup cornstarch

Combine the ingredients very well with a whisk. Pour into a mason jar with holes poked into the lid. Shake the powder inside a pillowcase or under the sheets, and wake up in the morning with renewed energy after a cool, peaceful night's sleep. When storing your jar, you can place a piece of plastic wrap under the lid so that the powder won't spill out of the jar. Store in a jar with a tight-fitting lid, in a cool, dark, dry area, for up to 3 months.

ACHE AND PAIN BATH RELIEVER

Once you have the flu, your body is in a lot of pain in the muscles and joints; sometimes it feels like it's in the bones themselves. This healing, soothing bath will help you feel like your old self, and the oils can help treat a myriad of symptoms. The all-natural healing benefits in this recipe are derived from the anti-inflammatory, antiseptic, decongestant, expectorant, and sudorific agents in these essential oils.

YIELD: 1 APPLICATION

4 drops tea tree (melaleuca) oil
3 drops lavender oil
2 drops lemon oil
2 drops cypress oil
1 tablespoon carrier oil
1 tablespoon milk (optional for adults,
    recommended for children)

While the bathwater is running, pour the essential oils and the carrier oil into the bath. Make sure that the water is not so hot as to cause the essential oils to dissipate. Oftentimes people add 1 tablespoon milk to the water; this will cause the essential oil to blend into the water and not float on top of the water. Soak in the water as long as you are comfortable. Store the remainder in a jar with a tight-fitting lid, in a cool, dark area, for up to 1 month.

MUSCLE MASSAGE

To help end the muscle aches and pains and make it through another day, use the essential oils in this recipe for their therapeutic analgesic, antibacterial, anti-inflammatory, antimicrobial, antispasmodic, and antiviral elements.

YIELD: 2 TO 6 APPLICATIONS

3 drops tea tree (melaleuca) oil
2 drops eucalyptus oil
2 drops lemon oil
1 ounce carrier oil

In a small container, drip the essential oils. Pour in the carrier oil and swirl to mix the oils. Rub the back, chest, and neck areas lightly with your fingertips or a soft cloth dipped into the mixture to ensure that the essential oils are distributed over the skin. You can also pour into a roll-on bottle and roll onto the desired area. Be sure not to get any into the eyes or sensitive areas. Store unused portion in a jar with a tight-fitting lid, in a cool, dark area, for up to 3 months.

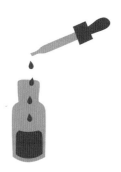

FUNGUS

Fungus germs lurk in public places and can be spread from person to person, especially if you go barefoot or share items, such as towels. Certain illnesses and allergies can cause fungus to sprout anywhere on the body. Fungus bacteria is prevalent among athletes and in crowded situations. Essential oils can reduce or eliminate the risk of a fungal infection, and work wonders in healing fungus once it attacks. Fungus infections can appear as red, itchy, patchy areas on the skin and can last for years. Candidiasis and celiac disease, among others, cause fungal attacks anywhere on the body, and the culprit is usually sugar, wheat, or a host of other foods. So stay away from that cupcake and turn to your essential oils.

Essential Oils: cinnamon, thyme, clove, tea tree (melaleuca), oregano, rosemary, lavender, myrrh, melissa, marjoram, lemongrass, lemon, cassia, clary sage, cypress, eucalyptus, helichrysum, grapefruit, geranium, fennel, wintergreen, chamomile, peppermint, patchouli, neem, and cedarwood

FUNKY FUNGUS RUB

These essential oils fight fungus and have many

healing effects that are beneficial to your whole body with their antifungal properties.

YIELD: 1 APPLICATION

1 drop clove oil
1 drop cinnamon oil
1 drop peppermint oil
1 teaspoon carrier oil

In a small container, drip the essential oils. Pour in the carrier oil and swirl to mix the oils. Rub the affected area lightly with your fingertips or a soft cloth dipped into the mixture to ensure that the essential oils are distributed over the skin. You can also pour into a roll-on bottle and roll onto the desired area. Be sure not to get any into the eyes or sensitive areas. If any of the mixture remains, store in a container with a tight-fitting lid in the refrigerator for up to 3 days.

FRESH AIR

Antifungal properties permeate the air and fight fungus wherever it resides in your home.

YIELD: 1 APPLICATION

4 drops peppermint oil
4 drops cinnamon oil
Water

Most diffusers come with directions for using essential oils. Add the manufacturer's recommended amount of water and the oils to the diffuser and run your delightful diffuser several times a day to receive the desired effect.

FUNGUS SPRAY

The essential oils in this spray bring quick relief to the itchy, painful fungus-infested area on your skin. Carry this in your purse for when you're out of town, or to use at the office. The healing antifungal properties of this recipe will help bring fungus to an end.

YIELD: 25 TO 50 SPRAYS PER 2-OUNCE BOTTLE

1 drop cinnamon oil
1 drop rosemary oil
1 drop lemon oil
2 ounces water

Combine the ingredients in a 2-ounce spray bottle and lightly spray the affected area. Allow to air dry. The essential oils will be absorbed into the skin by contact. Store in a spray bottle in a cool, dark area for up to 3 months.

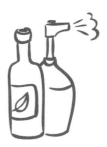

GERMS

Essential oils can assist in cleaning your home and keeping it as germ-free as possible. Many essential oils are natural germ fighters and can make a significant difference in preventing flu and other types of germs from entering our lives.

Essential Oils: tea tree (melaleuca), lemon, eucalyptus, and orange

GERM-KILLER POWDER

This germ-fighting powder will protect you while you sleep. These essential oils have therapeutic properties that can help guard you from many types of airborne illnesses. The antiviral, antiseptic, and antibacterial properties in this blend kill germs quickly.

YIELD: 10 TO 20 APPLICATIONS

3 drops tea tree (melaleuca) oil
3 drops orange oil
3 drops eucalyptus oil
¼ cup cornstarch

Combine all the ingredients together in a bowl, using a whisk. Place the mixture in a mason jar with holes poked into the lid. Shake the powder into a pillowcase or under the sheet as needed.

You can get a piece of plastic wrap and place it over the jar, under the lid, to keep the powder from spilling out when not in use. Store in a cool, dark, dry area for up to 3 months.

SUPER GERM-FIGHTING SPRAY

When everyone else is falling by the wayside with flu and viruses, you will have this secret weapon handy to spray away your family's fears of getting sick. These essential oils are some of the strongest in the world for protecting you against germs. This recipe is full of antibacterial, antibiotic, antifungal, anti-infectious, and antimicrobial properties to fight germs everywhere.

YIELD: 25 TO 50 SPRAYS PER 2-OUNCE BOTTLE

12 drops tea tree (melaleuca) oil
8 drops eucalyptus oil
5 drops lemon oil
2 ounces water

Combine the ingredients in a 2-ounce spray bottle and lightly spray the affected area. Allow to air dry. The essential oils will kill germs on contact and help keep the spread of those germs at bay. Store in the spray bottle in a cool, dark area for up to 3 months.

HAIR LOSS

There are numerous reasons why a person can suffer from hair loss. Alopecia is a disease that characteristically includes massive hair loss. Chemotherapy and some medications can also cause a person to lose their hair, in addition to old age, illness, drugs, heredity, chemicals, and various other factors. Essential oils can alleviate some hair loss in certain situations.

Essential Oils: ylang-ylang, sage, lavender, clary sage, lemon, peppermint, cedarwood, and rosemary

RESTORATIVE SHAMPOOS

The essential oils listed above are reported to re-grow hair after it begins falling out. A shampoo made with these oils, which contain antifungal, anti-inflammatory, and astringent properties, may help reduce issues that cause hair loss.

YIELD: 20 TO 40 APPLICATIONS

10 drops any one of the essential oils listed above, or 2 drops rosemary oil, 2 drops clary sage oil, 3 drops cypress oil, and 3 drops sandalwood oil
1 cup any shampoo

Add the essential oils to the shampoo. You may combine the oils, or try them one at a time. Stir to mix the oils with the shampoo before each use. Shampoo hair as usual. Store the remainder in bottle with a tight-fitting lid in a cool, dark area, for up to 3 months.

SCALP RESTORATIVE SPRAY

Spray this on your hair daily to stimulate the scalp and rejuvenate your hair to new life.

YIELD: 50 TO 100 SPRAYS PER 4-OUNCE BOTTLE

5 drops rosemary oil
5 drop lavender oil
4 ounces water

Combine the ingredients in a spray bottle and lightly spray the hair and scalp. Allow to air dry. The essential oils will be absorbed into the skin by contact and permeate the hair follicles. Store in the spray bottle in a cool, dark area for up to 3 months.

HANGOVER

The physical effects a person experiences after consuming a lot of alcohol is called a hangover. Usually the next day a person is disoriented, nauseous, and has digestive issues, a headache, and other uncomfortable side effects. People with hangovers often appear sick, they can't think straight, and they think they have great stories to tell. Essential oils can help a person recover from many of the ill effects of alcohol consumption.

Essential Oils: rosemary, rose, juniper, lemon, lavender, grapefruit, and sandalwood

I'LL NEVER DO THAT AGAIN BATH

When you swore you'd never do it again, yet . . . you did it again. Quell those feelings of illness with these restorative essential oils that have anti-inflammatory, antioxidant, antispasmodic, and digestive agents.

YIELD: 1 APPLICATION

2 drops lemon oil
2 drops lavender oil
2 drops sandalwood oil
3 drops rosemary oil
1 tablespoon carrier oil
1 tablespoon milk (optional for adults)

While the bathwater is running, pour the ingredients into the bath. Make sure that the water is not so hot as to cause the essential oils to dissipate. Oftentimes people add 1 tablespoon milk

to the water; this will cause the essential oil to blend into the water and not float on top. Soak in the water as long as you are comfortable.

HELP ME, PLEASE, MASSAGE

Feel like you wanna die? Ask your partner to rub down your back and neck with this essential oil blend and you will feel like facing the day with renewed vigor. The active agents in this blend contain analgesic, anti-inflammatory, and carminative properties to help you get back to normal.

YIELD: 4 TO 10 APPLICATIONS

3 drops rosemary oil
2 drops juniper oil
2 drops lavender oil
2 drops lemon oil
2 drops grapefruit oil
2 ounces carrier oil

In a small container, drip the essential oils. Pour in the carrier oil and swirl to mix the oils. Rub the back or neck area lightly with your fingertips or a soft cloth dipped into the mixture to ensure that the essential oils are distributed over the skin. You can also pour into a roll-on bottle and roll onto the desired area. Be sure not to get any into the eyes or sensitive areas. Store the remainder in a jar with a tight-fitting lid, in a cool, dark area, for up to 3 months.

SOBER AIR

This diffuse recipe will work wonders when you have a hangover. You'll feel better, and your house will smell great too! The ingredients in these oils, in part, are antispasmodic, nervine, and stomachic components that will have you back in party mode in no time.

YIELD: 1 APPLICATION

4 drops rose oil
3 drops lavender oil
2 drops lemon oil
2 drops sandalwood oil
Water

Most diffusers come with directions for using essential oils. Add the manufacturer's recommended amount of water and the oils to the diffuser and run your delightful diffuser several times a day to receive the desired effect.

HAY FEVER

When a person has a reaction to plant pollen, it is called hay fever, even though no fever is usually present. It produces coldlike symptoms and can last for days, or even weeks—at which point, you should see a doctor for diagnosis. Essential oils can vastly improve certain symptoms in most individuals. Many people in my family suffer from hay fever—sadly, we live in an area in Texas surrounded by hay fields! These are the essential oils that we use to help us get through those summer months.

Essential Oils: eucalyptus, tea tree (melaleuca), melissa, Roman chamomile, juniper, pine, rose, patchouli, niaouli, basil, peppermint, lemon, and lemongrass

UN-STOP ME SPRAY

This spray can be carried with you wherever you go. The essential oils in this spray are quite effective at clearing out the sinuses with their analgesic, antifungal, antimicrobial, and antiseptic properties. It is hay fever season right now, and my husband is using this spray every day to keep his hay fever at bay.

YIELD: 25 TO 50 SPRAYS PER 2-OUNCE BOTTLE

4 drops eucalyptus oil
4 drops lemon oil
2 ounces water

Combine the ingredients in a spray bottle and lightly spray yourself, the room, your car or anywhere you like. The essential oils will be absorbed into the skin by contact or by lungs if sprayed into the air. Store in the spray bottle in a cool, dark area for up to 3 months.

NO-WEEDS AIR

This great diffuse recipe will have you breathing like yourself in no time with these sinus-clearing essential oils. This blend contains analgesic, decongestant, and expectorant agents that work together to have you breathing easy, quickly.

YIELD: 1 APPLICATION

2 drops lemon oil
2 drops lemongrass oil
2 drops niaouli oil
1 drop patchouli oil
Water

Most diffusers come with directions for using essential oils. Add the manufacturer's recommended amount of water and the oils to the diffuser and run your delightful diffuser several times a day to receive the desired effect.

SINUS CLEARER

These essential oils provide you with a split-second remedy for that sinus headache. The therapeutic properties in these oils contain analgesic, antihistaminic, febrifuge, and sudorific elements.

YIELD: 1 APPLICATION

1 drop eucalyptus oil, or 1 drop melissa oil, or 1 drop peppermint oil

Place the drop of essential oil on a handkerchief or tissue, in the palm of your hand, or into an essential oil inhaler. Cup to your nose and inhale the aroma. Repeat several times daily or as needed.

HEADACHE

Pain or other symptoms in the head or neck area are often categorized as simply "headache." There are many possible reasons for pain in the head or neck; if symptoms persist, seek medical assistance to diagnose the cause. Healers have used the plants from which we extract essential oils for thousands of years to help reduce the throbbing, stabbing pain associated with headaches—even migraines.

Essential Oils: peppermint, cajeput, rosemary, basil, frankincense, clary sage, lemongrass, eucalyptus, chamomile, marjoram, lavender, ginger, clove, jasmine, thyme, sage, rose, grapefruit, bergamot, patchouli, and lemon

MAKE IT GO AWAY WASH

This is the perfect blend of essential oils to quickly and effectively banish pain while leaving behind a beautiful aroma. Its therapeutic properties—analgesic, anti-inflammatory, antispasmodic, and stimulating agents—will ease the pain quickly.

YIELD: 1 APPLICATION

7 drops lavender oil
5 drops eucalyptus oil
2 ounces water

Combine the ingredients in a bowl. With a soft washcloth, apply the mixture to the head, temples, and neck area and let air dry. Never apply to open wounds or near sensitive body parts. Use all of the mixture within a 24-hour period, and discard any remaining after that.

TEMPLE MASSAGE

The essential oils in this recipe have long been known to banish the headache blues. Massage it into your temples and the back of your neck and you will forget about your headache in no time. Cephalic, analgesic, nervine, and vasodilator properties will bring speedy relief.

YIELD: 1 APPLICATION

3 drops lavender oil

1 drop marjoram oil
1 drop clary sage oil
1 drop chamomile oil
1 teaspoon carrier oil

In a small container, drip the essential oils. Pour in the carrier oil and swirl to mix the oils. Rub the temples and back of neck area lightly with your fingertips or a soft cloth dipped into the mixture to ensure that the essential oils are distributed over the skin. You can also pour into a roll-on bottle and roll onto the desired area. Be sure not to get any into the eyes or sensitive areas. If any of the mixture remains, store in a container with a tight-fitting lid in the refrigerator for up to 3 days.

STRAIGHT TO THE BRAIN

Carry these essential oils in your purse and they will be ready at a moment's notice when you feel that headache trying to sneak its way in. These oils contain anti-inflammatory, tonic, and analgesic properties to help end the pain.

YIELD: 1 APPLICATION

1 drop lavender oil, or 1 drop frankincense oil, or 1 drop lemongrass oil, or 1 drop peppermint oil

Place the drop of essential oil on a handkerchief or tissue, in the palm of your hand, or in an essential oil inhaler. Cup to your nose and inhale the aroma. Repeat several times daily or as needed.

HEARING LOSS

Many people notice a loss of hearing over a period of time; it's generally associated with old age, but can also result from a host of illnesses. A physician can determine the cause of your hearing loss, and many times it can be corrected. Essential oils have helped in certain instances to correct or improve hearing loss. Never place essential oils directly into the ear—apply to the outer ear only.

Essential Oils: eucalyptus, fennel, white fir, geranium, helichrysum, and lavender

OUTER EAR RUB

This recipe includes essential oils known for their healing and pain-reducing properties. Rub around the outer ear to get the benefits. (Never place essential oils inside the ear.) The therapeutic properties that help alleviate ear pain are analgesic, antibacterial, antifungal, and anti-inflammatory.

Yield: 1 application

3 drops helichrysum oil
2 drops geranium oil
1 drop fennel oil
1 teaspoon carrier oil

In a small container, drip the essential oils. Pour in the carrier oil and swirl to mix the oils. Rub the outer ear area lightly with your fingertips or a soft cloth dipped into the mixture to ensure that the essential oils are distributed over the skin. You can also pour into a roll-on bottle and roll onto the desired area. Be sure not to get any into the eyes or sensitive areas. If any of the mixture remains, store in a container with a tight-fitting lid in the refrigerator for up to 3 days.

FROM MY NOSE TO MY EAR

This quick little recipe is made with essential oils believed to clear out the tubes causing your hearing loss and/or ear discomfort. The therapeutic properties in these oils are, in part, analgesic, antifungal, anti-inflammatory, bactericidal, and mucolytic. Never place essential oils inside the ear.

Yield: 1 application

1 drop eucalyptus oil, or 1 drop lavender oil

Place the drop of essential oil on a handkerchief or tissue, in the palm of your hand, or in an essential oil inhaler. Cup to your nose and inhale the aroma. Repeat several times daily or as needed.

HEARTBURN

When eating spicy food, many people experience pain or a burning sensation radiating from the chest up to the throat or neck. This is known in some instances as heartburn. Rubbing essential oils on the chest or throat can alleviate some of the symptoms of heartburn, and can often eradicate it all together. Heartburn can be indicative of other illnesses, so if symptoms persist, please contact a physician.

Essential Oils: black pepper, ginger, sandalwood, peppermint, eucalyptus, cardamom, basil, frankincense, lemon, Roman chamomile, and orange

THROAT RUB

I actually tried this yesterday after having heartburn for two days straight. After a couple of hours I thought, "Huh. My heartburn is gone." I love me some essential oils! The reliev-

ing agents at work in this recipe are antiemetic, anti-inflammatory, antispasmodic, and digestive properties.

YIELD: 2 TO 4 APPLICATIONS

2 drops eucalyptus oil
2 drops peppermint oil
1 drop fennel oil
1 drop frankincense oil
1 ounce carrier oil

In a small container, drip the essential oils. Pour in the carrier oil and swirl to mix the oils. Rub the lower abdomen area lightly with your fingertips or a soft cloth dipped into the mixture to ensure that the essential oils are distributed over the skin. You can also pour into a roll-on bottle and roll onto the desired area. Be sure not to get any into the eyes or sensitive areas. Store the remainder in a jar with a tight-fitting lid, in a cool, dark area for up to 3 months.

DRINK RELIEF

This quick remedy has been used for years due to its antispasmodic, detoxifying, and tonic healing properties.

YIELD: 1 TO 2 APPLICATIONS

1 drop lemon oil
4 ounces water

Ensure that your essential oil is safe for consumption and internal use and are clinical/therapeutic grade. Mix the oil with the water and drink slowly. Store unused portion in a jar with a tight-fitting lid, in a cool, dark area or the refrigerator, for up to 1 day.

CHEST MASSAGE

This relieving rub will have you feeling better in no time at all. These essential oils will work effectively and quickly with their inflammatory, carminative, digestive, and warming properties. Anyone suffering from heartburn can tell you that it is annoying, uncomfortable, and sometimes painful. This blend will have you feeling better, quickly.

YIELD: 4 TO 10 APPLICATIONS

2 drops eucalyptus oil
2 drops cardamom oil
2 drops orange oil
1 drop black pepper oil
2 ounces carrier oil

In a small container, drip the essential oils. Pour in the carrier oil and swirl to mix the oils. Rub the lower abdomen area lightly with your fingertips or a soft cloth dipped into the mixture to ensure that the essential oils are distributed over the skin. You can also pour into a roll-on bottle and roll onto the desired area. Be sure not to get any into the eyes or sensitive areas. Store the remainder in a jar with a tight-fitting lid, in a cool, dark area, for up to 3 months.

HEAT EXHAUSTION

This is a mild form of the more serious medical emergency condition of heat stroke, which results mainly from extended exposure to heat, usually from the sun. Essential oils can be used to cool down the body and give you some relief. Any significant rise in body temperature, especially in children and the elderly, requires immediate medical attention.

Essential Oils: peppermint, lavender

COOLDOWN RAG

The cooling, inflammatory, and invigorating properties in these essential oils will help you fight off that heat and bring cool relief. Place the cloth on the back of your neck or forehead and you will feel better immediately. This just feels so good after a day of mowing the lawn or any outdoor work.

YIELD: 1 APPLICATION

2 drops peppermint oil
1 drop lavender oil
1 wet cloth

Use gauze, linen, or any comfortable, clean cloth. Mix the ingredients, drip onto the cloth, and place over the affected area. Leave on until the cloth is no longer cool, then reapply as often as you want.

COLOR ME COOL

Inhaling the aroma of these essential oils instantly cools the brain and helps to alleviate the heat. The healing properties of these oils include analgesic, cooling, anti-inflammatory, and astringent agents.

YIELD: 1 APPLICATION

1 drop lavender oil
1 drop peppermint oil

Place the drops of essential oils on a handkerchief or tissue, in the palm of your hand, or in an essential oil inhaler. Cup to your nose and inhale the aroma. Repeat several times daily or as needed.

HEMORRHOIDS

Inflammation of the veins and tissues surrounding the anal area is painful when the membranes are swollen. Medical treatment can often bring much-needed relief to a person suffering from hemorrhoids, and essential oils and herbal rubs have been used for centuries to alleviate some of this suffering. Always consult with a physician if you are taking any medications, as these oils often have a countereffect on the medications.

Essential Oils: cypress, helichrysum, lavender, geranium, frankincense, peppermint, sandalwood, balsam, coriander, juniper, myrrh, patchouli, and yarrow

GET THOSE BASTARDS BATH TREATMENT

Hemorrhoids are ugly and a constant pain in the ass! Shrink them and alleviate the pain by soaking in this bath of healing essential oils with their anti-inflammatory, vasoconstrictor, and antiseptic properties.

YIELD: 1 APPLICATION

3 drops cypress oil
3 drops juniper oil
2 drops myrrh oil

1 drop sandalwood oil

1 drop balsam oil

2 tablespoons carrier oil

1 tablespoon milk (optional for adults,
*   recommended for children)*

While the bathwater is running, pour the ingredients into the bath. Make sure that the water is not so hot as to cause the essential oils to dissipate. Oftentimes people add 1 tablespoon milk to the water; this will cause the essential oil to blend into the water and not float on top of the water. Soak in the water as long as you are comfortable.

MIKE'S SHRINK 'EM BATH

My brother's hemorrhoids were so prevalent in his life that he named them. This recipe brought him much-needed relief and he took this bath often. The therapeutic properties in this all-natural blend include anti-inflammatory, analgesic, and antiseptic components.

YIELD: 1 APPLICATION

2 drops helichrysum oil

2 drops frankincense oil

2 drops lavender oil

2 drops cypress oil

2 tablespoons carrier oil

1 tablespoon milk (optional for adults,
*   recommended for children)*

As the bathwater is running, pour the ingredients into the bath. Make sure that the water is not so hot as to cause the essential oils to dissipate. Oftentimes people add 1 tablespoon milk to the water; this will cause the essential oil to blend into the water and not float on top. Soak in the water as long as you are comfortable.

HICCUPS

A catch in the diaphragm causes hiccups. This anomaly goes away on its own, but there are multiple "old wives' tales" about how to cure the hiccups—we're sure you've tried a few. BOO! Essential oils have been known to reduce the slight pain often associated with having the hiccups as well as to shorten their duration.

Essential Oils: dill, fennel, tarragon, peppermint, sandalwood, basil, and mandarin

STO-O-O-OP! DRINK

Give it a try! See if you can stop the hiccups with this drink and its anti-inflammatory benefits.

YIELD: 1 TO 2 APPLICATIONS

2 drops peppermint oil
4 ounces water

Ensure that your essential oil is safe for consumption and internal use and is clinical/therapeutic grade. Mix the oil and water and drink slowly. Store unused portion in a jar with a tight-fitting lid, in a cool, dark area or the refrigerator, for up to 1 day.

THROAT RUB

The essential oils from these plants have long been reputed to stop the hiccups with their antispasmodic elements. Rub it on and give it a try.

YIELD: 1 TO 2 APPLICATIONS

2 drops dill oil
1 drop basil oil
1 drop peppermint oil
1 tablespoon carrier oil

In a small container, drip the essential oils. Pour in the carrier oil and swirl to mix the oils. Rub the throat and chest area lightly with your fingertips or a soft cloth dipped into the mixture to ensure that the essential oils are distributed over the skin. You can also pour into a roll-on bottle and roll onto the desired area. Be sure not to get any into the eyes or sensitive areas. Store the remainder in a jar with a tight-fitting lid, in a cool, dark area, for up to 1 month.

BREATHE THE GOOD BREATH AIR

Run this blend of essential oils in your diffuser to rid yourself of the hiccups! The antispasmodic, anti-inflammatory, and digestive therapeutic properties of this recipe will work wonders, and your home will smell great at the same time.

YIELD: 1 APPLICATION

3 drops tarragon oil
2 drops peppermint oil
2 drops dill oil
2 drops mandarin oil
Water

Most diffusers come with directions for using essential oils. Add the manufacturer's recommended amount of water and the oils to the diffuser and run your delightful diffuser several times a day to receive the desired effect.

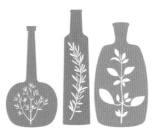

HIGH BLOOD PRESSURE

(Hypertension)

Following a well-balanced diet, exercising, and reducing stress are the greatest warriors for people suffering from high blood pressure. People have used the plants from which we extract these essential oils for thousands of years to assist in controlling blood pressure. However, high blood pressure can lead to a myriad of serious complications. Consult your physician to ensure that your medications do not counteract with the essential oils. Never use hyssop, sage, rosemary, or thyme if you have high blood pressure, as these oils are known to raise blood pressure.

Essential Oils: clary sage, ylang-ylang, marjoram, lavender, cassia, lime, frankincense, garlic, clove, eucalyptus, wintergreen, and lemon

SMELL ME MELLOW

This blend of essential oils will have your stress level reduced and your blood pressure down in no time. The stress-relieving recipe includes antidepressant, hypertensive, and euphoric properties.

Yield: 1 application

1 drop ylang-ylang oil
1 drop lavender oil
1 drop helichrysum oil
1 drop lemon oil
Water

Most diffusers come with directions for using essential oils. Add the manufacturer's recommended amount of water and the oils to the diffuser and run your delightful diffuser several times a day to receive the desired effect.

HIGH TO LOW RUB

This nice foot rub contains essential oils that will reduce your blood pressure and have you feeling great with its calming and hypotensive properties. The soles of the feet have been proven to absorb the oils and transport them to every cell in the body within minutes.

Yield: 1 application

2 drops helichrysum oil
2 drops frankincense oil
1 teaspoon carrier oil

In a small container, drip the essential oils. Pour in the carrier oil and swirl to mix the oils. Rub the soles of the feet lightly with your fingertips or a soft cloth dipped into the mixture to ensure that the essential oils are distributed over the skin. You can also pour into a roll-on bottle and roll onto the desired area. Be sure not to get any into the eyes or sensitive areas. Store the remainder in a jar with a tight-fitting lid, in a cool, dark area, for up to 3 days.

LOWER THAT PRESSURE BATH

Soak in this bath and let the stress and tension melt away. This recipe uses essential oils that are believed to lower blood pressure with hypotensive, sedative, and anti-inflammatory properties.

Yield: 1 application

3 drops lavender oil
2 drops frankincense oil
2 drops clary sage oil
1 tablespoon carrier oil
1 tablespoon milk (optional for adults,
*   recommended for children)*

While the bathwater is running, pour the essential oils and the carrier oil into the bath. Make sure that the water is not so hot as to cause the essential oils to dissipate. Oftentimes people add 1 tablespoon milk to the water; this will cause the essential oil to blend into the water and not float on top. Soak in the water as long as you are comfortable.

HIVES

Usually hives are an allergic reaction to food or environmental factors. You can complete an elimination test or get testing done by an allergist to determine what is causing the hives, which can even be a psychological issue. Essential oils can be used to soothe the skin and eliminate hives in some cases. Ensure through your physician that the oils won't counteract with the medications.

Essential Oils: peppermint, lavender, chamomile, tea tree (melaleuca), lemon, frankincense, coriander, myrrh, and helichrysum

ITCH-RELIEVING HIVE WASH

A cooling, relieving wash that helps hives go away instantly, the healing properties in this recipe include antiallergenic, antibiotic, analgesic, and anti-inflammatory agents.

Yield: 1 application

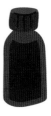

3 drops chamomile oil
2 drops lemon oil
2 drops lavender oil
2 drops helichrysum oil
3 tablespoons baking soda
1 cup water

Combine the ingredients in a bowl. With a soft washcloth, apply the mixture to the affected area and let air dry. Never apply to an open wound or near sensitive body parts. Use within 24 hours, then discard any remainder.

DAB IT ON

This is a quick fix you can carry in your purse or car to use at a moment's notice. Myrrh contains natural healing components with analgesic, antiseptic, astringent, cicatrisant, immune-stimulant, and anti-inflammatory properties.

YIELD: 1 APPLICATION

2 drops myrrh oil

Ensure that your essential oil is therapeutic or clinical grade before placing on the body, as essential oils can be very powerful. Myrrh essential oil can be placed directly on the skin (neat) without adding carrier oil to it. Apply with your fingertips or a soft cloth.

HORMONE IMBALANCE

Many essential oils contain natural hormones that, when rubbed on the body, can create a balance without using artificial hormones. I have had a hormone imbalance for several years due to menopause. I have noticed that days when I use these oils are much more productive than the days I don't use anything. My moods are stable and quite a bit more in tune while using these oils.

Essential Oils: cypress, lavender, clary sage, geranium, frankincense, neroli, rose, basil, bergamot, clove, ylang-ylang, wild orange, sandalwood, Roman chamomile, lime, lemon, grapefruit, and geranium

BALANCING POWDER

When PMS or menopause have you going a little crazy, sleep on this blend of essential oils to calm your mind and bring about a new attitude. A few of the sleep-inducing properties include antidepressant, nervine, and sedative elements.

YIELD: 10 TO 20 APPLICATIONS

3 drops wild orange oil

3 drops Roman chamomile oil

3 drops lavender oil

¼ cup cornstarch

Combine all the ingredients together in a bowl, using a whisk. Place in a mason jar with holes poked into the lid. Shake the powder into a pillowcase or under the sheet as needed. You can get a piece of plastic wrap and place it over the jar, under the lid, to keep the powder from spilling out when not in use. Store in a jar with a tight-fitting lid, in a cool, dark, dry area, for up to 3 months.

MASSAGE THE BITCH OUT OF ME

Yes, we've all been there. Even the sweetest of people can go a little psycho when their hormones are out of whack. These essential oils (not to mention the massage) will relax you and bring those hormones back into balance with their euphoric, aphrodisiac, hypotensive, nervine, and sedative properties.

YIELD: 2 TO 6 APPLICATIONS

3 drops cypress oil

3 drops lavender oil

2 drops frankincense oil

2 drops clary sage oil

1 ounce carrier oil

In a small container, drip the essential oils. Pour in the carrier oil and swirl to mix the oils. Rub the back, neck, and other areas lightly with your fingertips or a soft cloth dipped into the mixture to ensure that the essential oils are distributed over the skin. You can also pour into a roll-on bottle and roll onto the desired area. Be sure not to get any into the eyes or sensitive areas. Store unused portion in a jar with a tight-fitting lid, in a cool, dark area, for up to 3 months.

HORMONE-BALANCING SPRAY

When faced with a situation where you need to be on your best game, make the right choices, and keep a clear head, this essential oil spray will balance you out and keep you on the right track with its antidepressant, nervine, depurative, and uplifting properties.

YIELD: 50 TO 100 SPRAYS PER 4-OUNCE BOTTLE

6 drops neroli oil

4 drops rose oil

3 drops geranium oil

2 drops clove oil

4 ounces water

Combine the ingredients in a spray bottle and lightly spray the affected area. Allow to air dry. The essential oils will be absorbed into the skin by contact or by the lungs if sprayed into the air. Store in the spray bottle in a cool, dark area for up to 3 months.

HOT FLASHES

One horrible side effect of menopause is an overwhelming sense of heat that seems to start from the inside and burn through to your skin in one tenth of a second. This can range from an occasional burst of heat in some women to hundreds of times a day for other women. Essential oils can have a cooling effect, balance out the hormones, and sometimes decrease the instances of hot flashes. If you are on any medications, you must consult with your physician to ensure that the essential oils won't counteract your medications.

Essential Oils: peppermint, cypress, lemon, clary sage, and ylang-ylang

LORD HELP ME BATH

The cooling properties of these essential oils will help to alleviate and reverse the hot flashes you can experience with menopause. This bath was a lifesaver for me many times over.

YIELD: 1 APPLICATION

5 drops lemon oil

5 drops cypress oil

5 drops ylang-ylang oil

2 drops clary sage oil

1 tablespoon carrier oil

1 tablespoon milk

As the bathwater is running, pour the essential oils and the carrier oil into the bath. Make sure that the water is not so hot as to cause the essential oils to dissipate. Oftentimes people add 1 tablespoon milk to the water; this will cause the essential oil to blend into the water and not float on top. Soak in the water as long as you are comfortable.

COOL SHEETS LINEN POWDER

Stop those night sweats before they even start. Sprinkle this essential oil powder under your sheets and see if you don't have a night of cooling relief. The therapeutic properties in this recipe include analgesic, anti-inflammatory, cephalic, and cooling elements.

YIELD: 10 TO 20 APPLICATIONS

5 drops peppermint oil

4 drops lemon oil

4 drops clary sage oil

½ cup cornstarch

Combine the ingredients very well with a whisk. Pour into a mason jar with holes poked into the lid. Shake the powder inside a pillowcase or under the sheets, and wake up in the morning with renewed energy after a cool, peaceful night's sleep. When storing your jar, you can place a piece of plastic wrap under the lid so that the powder won't spill out of the jar. Store in a jar with a tight-fitting lid, in a cool, dark, dry area for up to 3 months.

COOLING RELIEF SPRAY

OMG! This spray is a must-have for women experiencing hot flashes. Handy to carry in your purse, or leave in an office desk. These cooling essential oils can bring down the heat stat with their astringent, cooling, tonic, and stimulating properties.

YIELD: 25 TO 50 SPRAYS PER 2-OUNCE BOTTLE

2 drops lemon oil
2 drops peppermint oil
2 ounces water

Combine the ingredients in a 2-ounce spray bottle and lightly spray the affected area. Allow to air dry. The essential oils will be absorbed into the skin by contact or by the lungs if sprayed into the air. Store in the spray bottle in a cool, dark area, for up to 3 months.

IMMUNITY BOOSTER

Our immune system is the best defense we have against all types of illnesses, from colds to cancer. Strengthening our immune system is paramount to maintaining optimal health, and essential oils have properties that are known immune boosters. Using these daily will help us to live better, healthier lives.

Essential Oils: thieves', tea tree (melaleuca), peppermint, myrtle, hyssop, thyme, geranium, rosemary, lemon, lavender, grapefruit, bergamot, and melissa

STRONG AIR

These protecting essential oils should be run all year round to help prevent colds, viruses, and the flu! Build up your immune system so that you can be at your optimal peak with the antiseptic, astringent, detoxifying, and immune-stimulating properties found in this blend.

YIELD: 1 APPLICATION

4 drops peppermint oil
3 drops hyssop oil

3 drops bergamot oil
2 drops lemon oil
Water

Most diffusers come with directions for using essential oils. Add the manufacturer's recommended amount of water and the oils to the diffuser and run your delightful diffuser several times a day to receive the desired effect.

SUPER IMMUNITY MUSCLES

These essential oil muscles work overtime to combat even the strongest opposing forces. Rub on when going out into public or when visiting sick friends for extra-powerful protection. The healing and protecting properties found in this recipe include antibacterial, antihistaminic, bactericidal, and disinfectant components.

YIELD: 4 TO 10 APPLICATIONS

4 drops tea tree (melaleuca) oil
3 drops thieves' oil
2 drops frankincense oil
2 drops melissa oil
2 drops grapefruit oil
2 ounces carrier oil

In a small container, drip the essential oils. Pour in the carrier oil and swirl to mix the oils. Rub the desired area lightly with your fingertips or a soft cloth dipped into the mixture to ensure that the essential oils are distributed over the skin. You can also pour into a roll-on bottle and roll onto the desired area. Be sure not to get any into the eyes or sensitive areas. Store the remainder in a jar with a tight-fitting lid, in a cool, dark area, for up to 3 months.

INHALE BUILDUP

Strong immune systems help us to kick the crap out of illnesses and disease. These powerful essential oils will help build the strong defense system you desire with their anti-inflammatory, antiseptic, and astringent properties.

YIELD: 1 APPLICATION

1 drop frankincense oil, or 1 drop tea tree (melaleuca) oil, or 1 drop lemon oil

Place the drop of essential oil on a handkerchief or tissue, in the palm of your hand, or in an essential oil inhaler. Cup to your nose and inhale the aroma. Repeat several times daily or as needed.

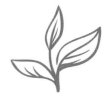

IMPETIGO

This condition is a skin infection caused by bacteria. Children are highly susceptible to impetigo, which is highly contagious and can be passed easily from child to child. Medical treatment can utilize medicines to treat this condition effectively, and the following essential oils are derived from plants and herbs that can complement a medical plan and prevent recurrence. Never use essential oils on children younger than four.

Essential Oils: frankincense, helichrysum, patchouli, geranium, oregano, lavender, tea tree (melaleuca), and myrrh

IMPETIGO BANDAGE

Children love bandages; they won't even notice you sneaking a drop or two of these safe but powerful essential oils into the mix. These oils heal and protect with their antibacterial, antibiotic, and anti-infectious therapeutic properties.

YIELD: 1 APPLICATION

2 drops lavender oil
2 drops tea tree (melaleuca) oil
1 drop myrrh oil
½ teaspoon carrier oil

Mix the ingredients well. Apply a few drops to a bandage or a piece of gauze with a cotton swab or your fingertips and secure to the site. Leave on for several hours or overnight. If any of the mixture remains, store in a container with a tight-fitting lid in the refrigerator for up to 3 days. If applying to a bandage or the skin, use a cotton swab or cotton ball to apply to avoid getting fingertips in the oil.

IMPETIGO RUB

When dealing with a very tender, painful sore, this rub can be lightly dabbed on to bring instant relief. Do not rub vigorously, as this could cause more pain. Do not apply oils to an open or gaping wound. The essential oils continue working for hours to promote healing and bring much relief to the patient with their anti-inflammatory, anti-infectious, and antibacterial components.

YIELD: 2 TO 6 APPLICATIONS

3 drops tea tree (melaleuca) oil
2 drops lavender oil
2 drops myrrh oil
1 drop helichrysum oil
1 ounce carrier oil

In a small container, drip the essential oils. Pour in the carrier oil and swirl to mix the oils. Rub the affected area lightly with your fingertips or a soft cloth dipped into the mixture to ensure that the essential oils are distributed over the skin. You can also pour into a roll-on bottle and roll onto the desired area. Be sure not to get any into the eyes or sensitive areas. Store the remainder in a jar with a tight-fitting lid, in a cool, dark area, for up to 1 month.

INFECTION-FIGHTING SPRAY

These essential oils are reported infection fighters. Keep this bottle handy to spray everywhere to get rid of infection and promote healing. The therapeutic properties at work in this blend include anti-inflammatory, antiseptic, and antiviral agents.

YIELD: 50 TO 100 SPRAYS PER 4-OUNCE BOTTLE

5 drops helichrysum oil
5 drops frankincense oil
5 drops lavender oil
4 ounces water

Combine the ingredients in a 4-ounce spray bottle and lightly spray the affected area or the air. Allow to air dry. The essential oils will be absorbed into the skin by contact or by the lungs if sprayed into the air, keeping germs at bay. Store in the spray bottle in a cool, dark area for up to 3 months.

INDIGESTION

Characterized by pain in the upper abdomen, indigestion is often accompanied by bloating, burning, nausea, and belching. Essential oils rubbed on the abdomen, throat, and chest can often relieve many of the symptoms of indigestion. If indigestion persists, consult a physician to ensure there are no underlying problems, issues, or illnesses.

Essential Oils: chamomile, fennel, ginger, peppermint, basil, cinnamon, thyme, rosemary, myrrh, marjoram, lavender, allspice, coriander, dill, basil, eucalyptus, angelica, frankincense, grapefruit, wild orange, cardamom, melissa, clary sage, hyssop, petitgrain, tangerine, and spikenard

EASY DRINK

This is just as good for you as ginger ale and has many healing benefits including analgesic, antiemetic, and stomachic properties.

YIELD: 1 TO 2 APPLICATIONS

1 drop ginger oil
4 ounces water

Ensure that your essential oil is safe for consumption and internal use and is clinical/therapeutic grade. Mix the oil and water and drink slowly. Store unused portion in a jar with a tight-fitting lid, in a cool, dark area or the refrigerator, for up to 1 day.

RUB ME BETTER

This chest rub is full of essential oils with indigestion-fighting properties that will have you feeling better all night long. The essential oils hard at work in this blend include anti-inflammatory, digestive, and stomachic agents to bring healing and relief to you quickly.

YIELD: 1 TO 2 APPLICATIONS

3 drops peppermint oil
2 drops lavender oil
1 drop ginger oil
1 tablespoon carrier oil

In a small container, drip the essential oils. Pour in the carrier oil and swirl to mix the oils. Rub the abdomen, chest, or back area lightly with your fingertips or a soft cloth dipped into the mixture to ensure that the essential oils are distributed over the skin. You can also pour into a roll-on bottle and roll onto the desired area. Be sure not to get any into the eyes or sensitive areas. Store the remainder in a jar with a tight-fitting lid, in a cool, dark area, for up to 1 month.

STOP IT RUB

This powerful blend of essential oils will stop that pain in its tracks. I like to make this recipe ahead of time when I know I am going to be eating the spicy foods that I love and crave. I always have it ready for when I am wallowing in my misery and paying for my cravings. But I love Mexican food and Italian food and the spicier the better! The therapeutic properties that help indigestion include stomachic, anti-inflammatory, carminative, and depurative components.

YIELD: 2 TO 6 APPLICATIONS

2 drops ginger oil
2 drops coriander oil
2 drops peppermint oil
2 drops chamomile oil
1 ounce carrier oil

In a small container, drip the essential oils. Pour in the carrier oil and swirl to mix the oils. Rub the chest, back, abdomen, or desired area lightly with your fingertips or a soft cloth dipped into the mixture to ensure that the essential oils are distributed over the skin. You can also pour into a roll-on bottle and roll onto the desired area. Be sure not to get any into the eyes or sensitive areas. Store unused portion in a jar with a tight-fitting lid, in a cool, dark area, for up to 3 months.

INFECTION

When bacteria, fungus, worms, or a virus invades the body, the body sometimes reacts with a fever trying to burn out the unwanted tiny guests. Infections can be slight, such as with a small cut, or can escalate to a medical emergency. If symptoms of infection persist, especially a fever, seek medical treatment. Ask your physician if these essential oils will conflict with any medications you are taking.

Essential Oils: thyme, rosemary, tea tree (melaleuca), clove, eucalyptus, basil, cinnamon, black pepper, grapefruit, garlic, ginger, coriander, camphor, bergamot, wild orange, peppermint, oregano, myrrh, marjoram, lime, lemon, geranium, cypress, lavender, and cassia

INFECTION BANDAGE

For a small cut or wound, this is the perfect recipe to place on a child's bandage. They won't even notice the essential oils or the powerful healing effect taking place under that cartoon bandage. The all-natural healing components of this recipe include analgesic, antibiotic, antifungal, anti-infectious, and anti-inflammatory properties.

YIELD: 1 APPLICATION

2 drops tea tree (melaleuca) oil
2 drops lavender oil
½ teaspoon carrier oil

Mix the ingredients well. Apply a few drops to a bandage or a piece of gauze with an eye dropper and secure to the site. Leave on for several hours or overnight. If any of the mixture remains, store in a container with a tight-fitting lid in the refrigerator for up to 3 days. If applying to bandage or skin, use a cotton swab, eye dropper, or cotton ball to apply to avoid getting fingertips in the oil.

INFECTION-FIGHTING AIR

Keep the air in your home or office germ free and antiseptic with this diffuser recipe that includes antibacterial, antifungal, and antimicrobial properties.

YIELD: 1 APPLICATION

3 drops eucalyptus oil
2 drops grapefruit oil
2 drops basil oil
1 drop cassia oil
Water

Most diffusers come with directions for using essential oils. Add the manufacturer's recommended amount of water and the oils to the diffuser and run your delightful diffuser several times a day to receive the desired effect.

GERM-KILLER SPRAY

These powerful infection- and germ-fighting essential oils will protect everything you touch. The germ-killing components are antiseptic, anti-infectious, anti-inflammatory, antibiotic, and antifungal properties. This is a powerful little protectant that I use during flu season and it really does the trick. Each of these essential oils alone is amazing, but combine them together and they are a force to be reckoned with.

YIELD: 50 TO 100 SPRAYS PER 4-OUNCE BOTTLE

10 drops tea tree (melaleuca) oil
4 drops clove oil
2 drops camphor oil
4 ounces water

Combine the ingredients in a 4-ounce spray bottle and lightly spray the room and the surrounding area. Allow to air dry. This spray will help in keeping germs on surfaces at bay. Store in a spray bottle in a cool, dark area for up to 3 months.

BE GONE INFECTION BATH

Soak in this bath and let these germ-fighting essential oils do their magic with their analgesic, antibacterial, antifungal, anti-inflammatory, and antimicrobial properties.

YIELD: 1 APPLICATION

6 drops tea tree (melaleuca) oil
6 drops eucalyptus oil
2 drops coriander oil
2 drops myrrh oil
1 tablespoon carrier oil
1 tablespoon milk (optional for adults, recommended for children)

While the bathwater is running, pour the ingredients into the bath. Make sure that the water is not so hot as to cause the essential oils to dissipate. Oftentimes people add 1 tablespoon milk to the water; this will cause the essential oil to blend into the water and not float on top. Soak in the water as long as you are comfortable.

INFLAMMATION

Usually a result of an infection, inflammation causes redness, swelling, pain, and sometimes loss of the use of the inflamed area. Essential oils can help reduce the symptoms of inflammation. Of course, any infection should always have medical treatment to ensure that the body can quickly recover. Ask your physician if these essential oils will conflict with any medications you are taking.

Essential Oils: helichrysum, frankincense, peppermint, lavender, myrrh, basil, eucalyptus, ginger, wintergreen, cassia, cinnamon, clove, geranium, lemon, jasmine, ylang-ylang, rose, and sandalwood

HOLLA RUB

These essential oils can reduce inflammation and speed up the healing process with their anti-inflammatory, anti-infectious, and antibacterial properties.

YIELD: 4 TO 10 APPLICATIONS

5 drops helichrysum oil
5 drops myrrh oil
5 drops lavender oil
5 drops rose oil
2 ounces carrier oil

In a small container, drip the essential oils. Pour in the carrier oil and swirl to mix the oils. Rub the desired area lightly with your fingertips or a soft cloth dipped into the mixture to ensure that the essential oils are distributed over the skin. You can also pour into a roll-on bottle and roll onto the desired area. Be sure not to get any into the eyes or sensitive areas. Store the remainder in a jar with a tight-fitting lid, in a cool, dark area, for up to 3 months.

HEALING HEALTHY RUB

This rub contains all the essential oils needed to promote healing and put a quick end to inflammation. The inflammatory fighting agents in this recipe include antimicrobial, astringent, antifungal, and anti-inflammatory therapeutic properties.

YIELD: 2 TO 6 APPLICATIONS

3 drops frankincense oil
3 drops cassia oil
1 drop clove oil
1 drop cinnamon oil
1 drop sandalwood oil
1 ounce carrier oil

In a small container, drip the essential oils. Pour in the carrier oil and swirl to mix the oils. Rub the desired area lightly with your fingertips or a soft cloth dipped into the mixture to ensure that the essential oils are distributed over the skin. You can also pour into a roll-on bottle and roll onto the desired area. Be sure not to get any into the eyes or sensitive areas. Store unused portion in a jar with a tight-fitting lid, in a cool, dark area, for up to 3 months.

INSECT BITES/ STINGS

These can be small harmless bites, such as those from mosquitoes, to painful and life-threatening ones, such as scorpion or spider bites. Caution and care must be used when treating any insect bite, and you must seek medical treatment when allergies to insect bites or respiratory issues arise. When a mosquito or an ant bites a person, it often leaves a small bump, itchiness, or a sting behind. For small insect bites that one is not allergic to, essential oils can provide immediate relief. If you suspect you are allergic to an insect and you get bitten, seek medical treatment immediately. There are numerous medications and instruments on the market today to assist a person with a life-threatening insect bite or sting.

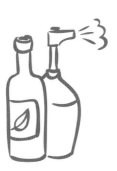

Essential Oils: lavender, tea tree (melaleuca), chamomile, peppermint, lemongrass, rosemary, basil, cinnamon, ylang-ylang, cajeput, niaouli, melissa, lime, lemon, eucalyptus, cypress, bergamot, clove, birch, pine, cedarwood, patchouli, citronella, orange, thyme, oregano, and helichrysum

BITE BANDAGE

This is a wonderful healing blend of essential oils to make ahead of time to dab on those inevitable bandages. Children will heal quickly and without the sting or burn that most store-bought chemical relievers contain. The healing properties in this recipe include antiallergenic, anti-inflammatory, and antiseptic agents.

YIELD: 1 APPLICATION

2 drops tea tree (melaleuca) oil
2 drops lavender oil
2 drops helichrysum oil
½ teaspoon carrier oil

Mix the ingredients well. Apply a few drops of the blend to a bandage or a piece of gauze with your fingertips or a cotton swab and secure to the site. Leave on for several hours or overnight. If any of the mixture remains, store in a container with a tight-fitting lid in the refrigerator for up to 3 days. If applying to a bandage or skin, use a cotton swab or cotton ball to apply to avoid getting fingertips in the oil.

BITE RELIEF ROLL-ON

This roll-on is handy to carry when camping or at the beach. Full of healing essential oils that will make your bug nibble disappear. The healing properties inherent in this blend include analgesic, antibiotic, anti-infectious, and anti-inflammatory components.

YIELD: 4 TO 10 APPLICATIONS

4 drops lavender oil
4 drops tea tree (melaleuca) oil
3 drops niaouli oil
3 drops chamomile oil
2 ounces carrier oil

Place the ingredients in a roll-on bottle. Roll around the site of the bite. Store the remainder in a jar with a tight-fitting lid, in a cool, dark area, for up to 3 months, or leave in the roll-on bottle in upright position.

BAD BUG-BITE BATH

When one of my grandsons was covered in mosquito bites after playing outside in the dark, I added these essential oils to his bath and he was instantly in heaven due to their analgesic, antibacterial, anti-inflammatory, and antiseptic therapeutic properties.

YIELD: 1 APPLICATION

5 drops lemongrass oil
4 drops rosemary oil
3 drops helichrysum oil
1 tablespoon carrier oil
1 tablespoon milk (optional for adults, recommended for children)

While the bathwater is running, pour the ingredients into the bath. Make sure that the water is not so hot as to cause the essential oils to dissipate. Oftentimes people add 1 tablespoon milk to the water; this will cause the essential oil to blend into the water and not float on top. Soak in the water as long as you are comfortable.

BITE/STING BANDAGE

This recipe is perfect for children: they love bandages and won't even notice that you have put a drop or two of this great healer on it first. These essential oils have long been known to bring relief to bug bites and stings with the curative properties of cicatrisant, detoxifying, and disinfectant compounds.

YIELD: 1 APPLICATION

2 drops tea tree (melaleuca) oil
1 drop lavender oil
1 drop peppermint oil
½ teaspoon carrier oil

Mix the ingredients well. Apply a few drops

of the ingredients to a bandage or a piece of gauze and secure to the site. Leave on for several hours or overnight. If any of the mixture remains, store in a container with a tight-fitting lid in the refrigerator for up to 3 days. If applying to a bandage or skin, use a cotton swab, eye dropper, or cotton ball to apply to avoid getting fingertips in the oil.

Insect Repellant

Many people prefer natural insect repellants in lieu of chemical-laden products bought at the store. Insect repellants are easy to make and are safe for children and the elderly. Here in Texas, if we want to sit outside on our porches in the evening, we don't have a choice. We must use something that will get rid of those varmints. Essential oil repellant works wonderfully—and smells good, too.

SPRAY IT IF YOU GOT IT!

This is a great spray to use on your clothing, furniture, and outdoor areas. Insects hate this smell and will stay away from you. Citronella is loaded with insect-repelling and vermifugal properties.

YIELD: 25 TO 50 SPRAYS PER 2-OUNCE BOTTLE

10 drops citronella oil

10 drops eucalyptus oil

6 drops geranium oil

1 ounce rubbing alcohol or vodka

2 ounces water

Combine the ingredients in a 2-ounce spray bottle and lightly spray the whole room area. This is safe enough to spray where people are sitting. Shake well before each use. Store in the spray bottle in a cool, dark area for up to 3 months.

SWELL REPEL

The herbs that these essential oils are derived from have been planted for years as bug deterrents. Now you can have a spray that does all of the work for you and keeps those pesky bugs at a distance. The essential oils listed in this recipe contain insect-repelling components that make it a powerful blend. Here in Texas, we have a bug epidemic each summer and this spray is great to use when you don't want to douse yourself in chemicals to keep them away.

YIELD: 50 TO 100 SPRAYS PER 4-OUNCE BOTTLE

4 drops lemongrass oil

4 drops thyme oil

4 drops lavender oil

4 drops peppermint oil

4 drops citronella oil

4 ounces water

Combine the ingredients in a 4-ounce spray bottle and lightly spray the whole body wherever skin is exposed. Allow to air dry. Store in the spray bottle in a cool, dark area for up to 3 months.

KEEP THEM OFF THE BED POWDER

This is a good one to take with you on camping trips. Just a little sprinkle under the sheets is enough to get those critters scampering far away from you.

YIELD: 10 TO 20 APPLICATIONS

3 drops peppermint oil

3 drops citronella oil

3 drops lavender oil

3 drops thyme oil

¼ cup cornstarch

Combine the ingredients very well with a whisk. Pour into a mason jar with holes poked into the lid. Shake the powder inside a pillowcase or un-

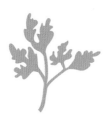

der the sheets, and wake up in the morning with renewed energy after a cool, peaceful night's sleep. When storing your jar, you can place a piece of plastic wrap under the lid so that the powder won't spill out of the jar. Store in a jar with a tight-fitting lid, in a cool, dark, dry area, for up to 3 months.

INSECT-REPELLANT SPRAY

I live in the country in Texas, and the spiders and beetles are rampant in July and August. I keep this by my bed because not only does it smell good to me, but as an added bonus the insects hate it and run away from the natural bug-repelling chemicals in this blend.

YIELD: 25 TO 50 SPRAYS PER 2-OUNCE BOTTLE

5 drops peppermint oil

3 drops rosemary oil

2 drops basil oil

2 drops thyme oil

2 ounces water

Combine the ingredients in a 2-ounce spray bottle and lightly spray the bed and floor area. Allow to air dry. This little mixture will work all night long in protecting your bed and home from those tiny invaders. Store in the spray bottle in a cool, dark area for up to 3 months.

ANT-REPELLANT SPRAY

Ants hate the smell and taste of peppermint oil. Use this spray around your windows and doors to keep those annoying little critters outside where they belong.

YIELD: 25 TO 50 SPRAYS PER 2-OUNCE BOTTLE

10 drops peppermint oil
10 drops rosemary oil
2 ounces water

Combine the ingredients in a 2-ounce spray bottle and lightly spray the ant-infested areas. Allow to air dry. The spray works night and day to protect your home. Store in a spray bottle in a cool, dark area for up to 3 months.

FLY-REPELLANT SPRAY

Each of these essential oils is a known enemy of flies. Spray your porch, chair, or wherever you and your friends are gathering. It's a great one to use at picnics.

YIELD: 25 TO 50 SPRAYS PER 2-OUNCE BOTTLE

7 drops peppermint oil
7 drops lavender oil
5 drops rosemary oil
2 ounces water

Combine the ingredients in a 2-ounce spray bottle and lightly spray the affected area. Allow to air dry. The essential oils will deter any fly that dares to get next to you or your picnic. Store in the spray bottle in a cool, dark area for up to 3 months.

SCORPION-REPELLANT SPRAY

The one essential oil known to repel scorpions is basil oil. If your home is infested with these dangerous, painful bugs (I really think they are tiny animals!), use this spray to run 'em out.

YIELD: 25 TO 50 SPRAYS PER 2-OUNCE BOTTLE

25 drops basil oil
2 ounces water

Combine the ingredients in a 2-ounce spray bottle and lightly spray the affected area. Allow to air dry. Scorpions hate this smell and will relocate to another place besides your home. Store in the spray bottle in a cool, dark area for up to 3 months.

MOSQUITO-REPELLANT SPRAY

Mosquitoes will turn around and fly away if they smell these essential oils. I like to spray this on my body before I go outside, and I also spray the chair I am going to sit in. This works very well on those spring nights when you just gotta be out on the porch.

YIELD: 25 TO 50 SPRAYS PER 2-OUNCE BOTTLE

10 drops lavender oil

10 drops lemongrass oil

2 ounces water

Combine the ingredients in a 2-ounce spray bottle and lightly spray the affected area. Allow to air dry. Store in the spray bottle in a cool, dark area for up to 3 months.

SPIDER-REPELLANT SPRAY

Oooh . . . I hate them! I will wear this, spray it on my bed, spray it on the toilet, and use it everywhere I am afraid a spider will show up in the middle of the night. Peppermint has been used for thousands of years as a spider repellant. We are lucky that now we have the oil from peppermint and we don't have to grow the plant under our beds!

YIELD: 25 TO 50 SPRAYS PER 2-OUNCE BOTTLE

25 drops peppermint oil

2 ounces water

Combine the ingredients in a spray bottle and lightly spray the affected area. Allow to air dry. Store in the spray bottle in a cool, dark area for up to 3 months.

INSOMNIA

Insomnia is rampant in the Western world. Stress, overwork, restless leg syndrome, illness, worry, and a host of other problems invade the mind and body when trying to sleep. Essential oils can work wonders on a person trying to get a good night's sleep in order to prepare for the day ahead.

Essential Oils: chamomile, lavender, bergamot, clary sage, marjoram, rose, sandalwood, ylang-ylang, petitgrain, mandarin, spikenard, vetiver, valerian, thyme, tangerine, yarrow, peppermint, frankincense, jasmine, basil, sage, melissa, and neroli

SLEEPY AIR TIME

This essential oil recipe turns those overly anxious, repetitive thoughts going through your head to dreams of beaches and comfort. Try this one before you go to bed tonight. This recipe contains properties such as sedative, aphrodisiac, and nervine agents.

YIELD: 1 APPLICATION

6 drops bergamot oil

4 drops lavender oil

4 drops frankincense oil

2 drops rose oil
Water

Most diffusers come with directions for using essential oils. Add the manufacturer's recommended amount of water and the oils to the diffuser and run your delightful diffuser an hour or two before bedtime to receive the desired effect.

DREAMTIME MASSAGE

The massage will help you to drift off and relax, but when coupled with this recipe you will find yourself dreaming of peaceful scenarios with abandon. The essential oils in this recipe contain sedative, tranquilizing, and relaxing agents.

YIELD: 4 TO 10 APPLICATIONS

4 drops lavender oil
3 drops clary sage oil
2 drops jasmine oil
2 drops ylang-ylang oil
2 ounces carrier oil

In a small container, drip the essential oils. Pour in the carrier oil and swirl to mix the oils. Rub the back, chest, neck, or temple area lightly with your fingertips or a soft cloth dipped into the mixture to ensure that the essential oils are distributed over the skin. You can also pour into a roll-on bottle and roll onto the desired

area. Be sure not to get any into the eyes or sensitive areas. Store the remainder in a jar with a tight-fitting lid, in a cool, dark area, for up to 3 months.

NIGHTY-NIGHT BATH

This recipe for your bedtime bath is loaded with essential oils that will have you struggling to stay awake long enough to make it to the bed. The therapeutic properties responsible for those slumber-inducing agents are nervine, sedative, and antidepressant.

YIELD: 1 APPLICATION

5 drops mandarin oil
5 drops petitgrain oil
4 drops chamomile oil
1 tablespoon carrier oil
1 tablespoon milk (optional for adults,
*   recommended for children)*

While the bathwater is running, pour the ingredients into the bath. Make sure that the water is not so hot as to cause the essential oils to dissipate. Oftentimes people add 1 tablespoon milk to the water; this will cause the essential oil to blend into the water and not float on top. Soak in the water as long as you are comfortable.

IBS
(Irritable Bowel Syndrome)

Allergies to foods, autoimmune disorders, and other ailments are often diagnosed as IBS, which is marked by chronic pain in the abdomen. Oftentimes, IBS symptoms can be alleviated by externally applying essential oils to reduce bloating, pain, and nausea. Consult a medical professional to ensure that nothing more serious is at the root of the pain.

Essential Oils: aloe vera, ginger, thyme, oregano, geranium, frankincense, peppermint, clove, and fennel

DRINK RELIEF

The plants that these essential oils are derived from have been used since the beginning of time to relieve stomach and intestinal pain. The therapeutic properties in these essential oils contain analgesic, antiemetic, carminative, and antispasmodic components.

Yield: 1 to 2 applications

1 drop ginger oil
1 drop peppermint oil
4 ounces water

Ensure that your essential oils are safe for consumption and internal use and are clinical/therapeutic grade. Mix the oils with the water and drink slowly. Store unused portion in a jar with a tight-fitting lid, in a cool, dark area or the refrigerator, for up to 1 day.

TUMMY TERROR RUB

This rub will do the trick by alleviating pain in the abdomen so that you can live your life to the fullest. These essential oils work well in reducing pain with their anesthetic, analgesic, and anti-inflammatory properties, to name a few.

Yield: 2 to 6 applications

2 drops peppermint oil
2 drops frankincense oil
2 drops geranium oil
1 drop oregano oil
2 tablespoons carrier oil

In a small container, drip the essential oils. Pour in the carrier oil and swirl to mix the oils. Rub the abdomen or desired area lightly with your fingertips or a soft cloth dipped into the mixture to ensure that the essential oils are distributed over the skin. You can also pour into a roll-on bottle and roll onto the desired area. Be sure not to get any into the eyes or sensitive areas. Store unused portion in a jar with a tight-fitting lid, in a cool, dark area, for up to 3 months.

JET LAG

When traveling, especially between continents, jet lag makes many of us miss a day of our vacations in order to sleep and "catch up." It is a lethargic, tired, exhausted feeling that persists for many hours or even days. There are many essential oils that can energize you and specifically reduce your time spent in the jet lag fog.

Essential Oils: geranium, peppermint, rosemary, basil, grapefruit, bergamot, neroli, vetiver, and lavender

MAKE THIS NAP COUNT POWDER

Make your nap in Paris count as an entire night with the relaxing sleep you'll get with this powder. It's easy to carry in your luggage and you can use it each night so that you'll rest easy and wake up refreshed. The sedative and nervine properties in this recipe work together to relax and calm you so you can wake fully rejuvenated.

YIELD: 10 TO 20 APPLICATIONS

3 drops lavender oil
3 drops neroli oil
3 drops vetiver oil
¼ cup cornstarch

Combine the ingredients very well with a whisk. Pour into a mason jar with holes poked into the lid. Shake the powder inside a pillowcase or under the sheets, and wake up in the morning with renewed energy after a cool, peaceful night's sleep. When storing your jar, you can place a piece of plastic wrap under the lid so that the powder won't spill out of the jar. Store in a jar with a tight-fitting lid, in a cool, dark, dry area, for up to 3 months.

CATCH ME UP SPRAY

When you don't have time for a nap, rejuvenate yourself with this refreshing spray to help get you through the next few hours feeling refreshed and vibrant. This little spray bottle is easy to transport in your luggage, and the energetic components in it contain tonic, antidepressant, and restorative stimulating properties.

YIELD: 50 TO 100 SPRAYS PER 4-OUNCE BOTTLE

4 drops geranium oil
4 drops vetiver oil
4 drops neroli oil
4 drops basil oil
4 ounces water

Combine the ingredients in a 4-ounce spray bottle and lightly spray the affected area. Allow to air dry. The essential oils will be absorbed into the skin by contact or by the lungs if sprayed into the air. Store in the spray bottle in a cool, dark area for up to 3 months.

TIME LEAP DRINK

To help you with that sometimes-nauseated feeling that accompanies jet lag, this recipe contains detoxifying and antispasmodic elements.

YIELD: 1 TO 2 APPLICATIONS

1 to 2 drops lemon oil
4 ounces water

Ensure that your essential oil is safe for consumption and internal use and is clinical/therapeutic grade. Mix the oil and water and drink slowly. Store unused portion in a jar with a tight-fitting lid, in a cool, dark area or the refrigerator, for up to 1 day.

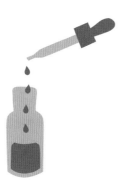

JOINT PAIN

The elbows, knees, hips, wrists, and ankles are most commonly affected by joint pain, but any joint in the body can have pain in it. The causes of joint pain are limitless, from arthritis to overwork and exhaustion. Essential oils can bring relief to those areas and calm that achy, sore feeling.

Essential Oils: birch, cypress, lavender, frankincense, chamomile, rosemary, clove, aloe vera, eucalyptus, oregano, wintergreen, cypress, fir, ginger, juniper, marjoram, peppermint

JOINT BATH SALTS

For centuries, people have relied on salt baths to work out the soreness in their joints by visiting the shores of distant seas to soak in the saltwater. These essential oils double the relief with the healing and therapeutic properties of analgesic, anti-inflammatory, and antispasmodic components.

YIELD: 5 TO 6 APPLICATIONS

7 drops ginger oil
7 drops juniper berry oil
7 drops frankincense oil
2 tablespoons carrier oil

3 cups salts (pink Himalayan salt, sea salt, or
Epsom salts)
1 tablespoon milk (optional for adults,
recommended for children)

Add the oils to the salt. Stir until the mixture is well blended. Put in a jar with a lid. Let sit for 24 hours and stir again. Do not make the bathwater too hot, as the oils will dissipate. Do not add the salts when the water is running, but add ½ cup of the bath salt mixture and the milk to the water as you get into the tub. Oftentimes people add 1 tablespoon milk to the water; this will cause the essential oil to blend into the water and not float on top. Store the remainder in a jar with a tight-fitting lid, in a cool, dark area, for up to 3 months.

SUPER PAIN REMEDY

A super rub that works fast and has long-lasting effects, the essential oils with pain-reducing components in this blend have analgesic, anti-inflammatory, antispasmodic, and antirheumatic therapeutic properties. This is great for those of us old geezers whose joints ache when the weather changes.

YIELD: 1 TO 2 APPLICATIONS

4 drops fir oil
2 drops rosemary oil

2 drops frankincense oil
1 tablespoon carrier oil

In a small container, drip the essential oils. Pour in the carrier oil and swirl to mix the oils. Rub the joints or desired area lightly with your fingertips or a soft cloth dipped into the mixture to ensure that the essential oils are distributed over the skin. You can also pour into a roll-on bottle and roll onto the desired area. Be sure not to get any into the eyes or sensitive areas. Store the remainder in a jar with a tight-fitting lid, in a cool, dark area, for up to 1 month.

ACHE RELIEF BATH

Rest those sore bones, joints, and muscles in this bath. This recipe contains analgesic, anti-inflammatory, and antioxidant agents, perfect for alleviating pain.

YIELD: 1 APPLICATION

7 drops aloe vera
5 drops chamomile oil

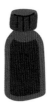

2 drops ginger oil

2 drops cypress oil

2 drops fir oil

1 tablespoon carrier oil

1 tablespoon milk (optional for adults, recommended for children)

While the bathwater is running, pour the essential oils and the carrier oil into the bath. Make sure that the water is not so hot as to cause the essential oils to dissipate. Oftentimes people add 1 tablespoon milk to the water; this will cause the essential oil to blend into the water and not float on top. Soak in the water as long as you are comfortable.

KNEE INJURY/PAIN

We need our knees! Knee pain must not be ignored and should be treated by a doctor. Essential oils can reduce the achy, sharp pains often suffered by those with "bad knees." Baths, rubs, and massages are the best treatment besides the treatment prescribed by your physician or rehab trainer. Never take any essential oils without first consulting with your physician to ensure the oils do not conflict with your medications.

Essential Oils: lavender, lemongrass, frankincense, helichrysum, white fir, oregano, eucalyptus, marjoram, peppermint, cypress, clove, cinnamon, and wintergreen

KNEE RUB

These essential oils are great to rub on your knees before you go to work or school. The mixture smells great and has energizing properties as well as anti-inflammatory, antispasmodic, and analgesic healing benefits.

Yield: 2 to 6 applications

2 drops peppermint oil

2 drops frankincense oil

2 drops lemon oil

1 drop helichrysum oil

1 ounce carrier oil

In a small container, drip the essential oils. Pour in the carrier oil and swirl to mix the oils. Rub the knees or desired area lightly with your fingertips or a soft cloth dipped into the mixture to ensure that the essential oils are distributed over the skin. You can also pour into a roll-on bottle and roll onto the desired area. Be sure not to get any into the eyes or sensitive areas. Store unused portion in a jar with a tight-fitting lid, in a cool, dark area, for up to 3 months.

LARYNGITIS

There are many ailments, from colds to vocal cord damage, that can cause laryngitis. Usually it is mild and can be treated with an over-the-counter medication or with a gargle. If laryngitis persists more than a week, it could be indicative of something more serious and you should visit your physician. Essential oils used in gargles can lessen the pain and hoarseness associated with laryngitis, but you must ensure that they can be taken orally.

Essential Oils: myrrh, frankincense, thyme, lavender, eucalyptus, sage, clary sage, benzoin, cajeput, geranium, niaouli, black pepper, rosemary, chamomile, tea tree (melaleuca), sandalwood, lemon, cinnamon, and clove

LIN'S GARGLE

Lin, my daughter, uses this remedy when she begins losing her voice after her bouts of bronchitis. It is quick and very effective with its antibacterial, antibiotic, and anti-inflammatory therapeutic properties.

YIELD: 1 TO 2 APPLICATIONS

1 drop rosemary oil
1 drop tea tree (melaleuca) oil
4 ounces water

Be sure that the oils you use are specifically labeled that they can be taken internally. Combine the oils and water. Swish in the mouth or gargle, then spit it out. Store unused portion in a jar with a tight-fitting lid, in a cool, dark area or the refrigerator, for up to 1 day.

THROAT RUB

These essential oils will help to restore your voice, alleviate pain, and relax your throat muscles with their analgesic, antibacterial, anti-inflammatory, and antiviral components.

YIELD: 1 APPLICATION

1 drop eucalyptus oil
1 drop lavender oil
1 drop lemon oil
1 drop frankincense oil
1 teaspoon carrier oil

In a small container, drip the essential oils. Pour in the carrier oil and swirl to mix the oils. Rub the outer throat and jaw area lightly with your fingertips or a soft cloth dipped into the mixture to ensure that the essential oils are distributed over the skin. You can also pour into a roll-on bottle and roll onto the desired area. Be sure not to get any into the eyes or sensitive areas. If any of the mixture remains, store in a container with a tight-fitting lid in refrigerator for up to 3 days.

LARYNGITIS DIFFUSER

This diffuse recipe has the essential oils needed to relax and give your throat muscles a break. The anti-inflammatory, bactericidal, analgesic, and stimulating agents work to bring you pain relief.

YIELD: 1 APPLICATION

4 drops lavender oil
3 drops eucalyptus oil
2 drops chamomile oil
2 drops myrrh oil
Water

Most diffusers come with directions for using essential oils. Add the manufacturer's recommended amount of water and the oils to the diffuser and run your delightful diffuser several times a day to receive the desired effect.

LICE

Those stinking little bugs that get in the kids' hair at school and hop from kid to kid are harder than anything to get rid of! Everybody hates lice. They are a pain and a chore to eradicate. And you must rid your home of every last one of them or they will rapidly multiply and infect your family again. Essential oils have been proven effective at ridding homes and people of lice without the chemicals that are in most lice shampoos today.

Essential Oils: tea tree (melaleuca), thyme, lavender, and pine

LICE CONDITIONER

I hate lice. My daughters had very long, thick hair and we would use this when they would come home from school with "the note." I loved using something on them that had absolutely no chemicals and was beneficial to them in every way.

YIELD: 1 TO 2 APPLICATIONS

4 drops tea tree (melaleuca) oil
2 drops thyme oil
2 drops pine oil
2 ounces coconut oil

Mix the ingredients and apply 1 teaspoon to the head and massage throughout the hair. Wrap with a towel or plastic wrap (do not cover the face with the plastic wrap) and leave on the head for 1 hour. Rinse and repeat 3 times in one day. After 7 days repeat the entire process to kill any eggs that have hatched. Be sure to wash all bedding and clothing each time.

LICE SPRAY

I would spray this everywhere in my home when I heard that there was a lice outbreak at school. Lice hate these essential oils and will not survive them!

YIELD: 50 TO 100 SPRAYS PER 4-OUNCE BOTTLE

5 drops tea tree (melaleuca) oil
5 drops lavender oil
5 drops pine oil
4 ounces water

Mix the ingredients in a 4-ounce spray bottle and spray the area throughout the week. During a lice infestation of your home, spray bedding, carpets, and furniture where lice thrive. Store in the spray bottle in a cool, dark area for up to 2 weeks.

LICE-PROTECTANT SHAMPOO

This recipe is easy to use and make. It protects your children 24-7 when lice are being transferred from child to child at school.

YIELD: 3 MONTH'S SUPPLY

20 drops lavender oil
1 bottle shampoo

Mix the essential oil into the shampoo and use as normal to protect your hair from lice looking for a home. Shake well before each use. Store in the shampoo bottle with a tight-fitting lid in a cool, dark area.

LOW BLOOD PRESSURE
(Hypotension)

When the blood pumping from the arteries is at a low rate, that's low blood pressure. Medications can be prescribed if other symptoms are present and it is ongoing. Check with your physician to ensure that these essential oils won't clash with your current medications.

Essential Oils: rose, cypress, lime, geranium, lemon, rosemary, helichrysum, sage, peppermint, pine, black pepper, benzoin, ginger, neroli, coriander, cypress, marjoram, eucalyptus, hyssop, and ylang-ylang

LOW TO HIGH RUB

The essential oils in this recipe will get you feeling back to normal with their restorative, stimulant, and hypertensive properties. Never use rosemary essential oil if you are pregnant.

YIELD: 2 TO 6 APPLICATIONS

2 drops cypress oil
2 drops rosemary oil
1 drop helichrysum oil
1 drop marjoram oil
1 ounce carrier oil

In a small container, drip the essential oils. Pour in the carrier oil and swirl to mix the oils. Rub the chest, neck, or back area lightly with your fingertips or a soft cloth dipped into the mixture to ensure that the essential oils are distributed over the skin. You can also pour into a roll-on bottle and roll onto the desired area. Be sure not to get any into the eyes or sensitive areas. Store unused portion in a jar with a tight-fitting lid, in a cool, dark area, for up to 3 months.

WHAT'S MY AIR PRESSURE?

This diffuser contains essential oils that will have your heart pumping and give you an all-over feeling of well-being. This recipe contains a blend that has hypertensive, tonic, and restorative properties.

YIELD: 1 APPLICATION

2 drops cypress oil
2 drops ylang-ylang oil
2 drops lavender oil
2 drops geranium oil
Water

Most diffusers come with directions for using essential oils. Add the manufacturer's recommended amount of water and the oils to the diffuser and run your delightful diffuser several times a day to receive the desired effect.

FOOT PRESSURE

This foot rub will get your heart rate up and give you energy at the same time. These essential oils contain hypertensive and restorative properties.

YIELD: 1 APPLICATION

2 drops marjoram oil
1 drop lemon oil
1 drop rosemary oil
½ teaspoon carrier oil

Combine the ingredients and rub into the soles of the feet as often as needed. The feet absorb essential oils and carry them to every cell in the body in a matter of minutes. If any of the mixture remains, store in a container with a tight-fitting lid in the refrigerator for up to 3 days.

MENOPAUSE

The horror that no one warned you about! Menopause affects every area of a woman's body and life. Hot flashes, night sweats, skin issues, depression, mood swings, slowing metabolism, and the list goes on. There are several essential oils that can help with every one of the issues that menopause brings. Ensure with your physician that the essential oils will not conflict with your medications.

Essential Oils: clary sage, cypress, geranium, neroli, fennel, Roman chamomile, bergamot, ylang-ylang, jasmine, rose, anise, lavender, angelica, coriander, and sage

MENOPAUSE BATH SALTS

Menopause is not taken lightly by anyone going through it. Use the essential oils in this recipe to calm you down and bring your emotions under control with their calming, antidepressant, and nervine properties.

YIELD: 5 TO 6 APPLICATIONS

7 drops anise oil
7 drops angelica essential oil
7 drops Roman chamomile oil
2 tablespoons carrier oil
3 cups salts (pink Himalayan salt, sea salt, or Epsom salts)
1 tablespoon milk (optional)

Add the oils to the salt. Stir until the mixture is well blended. Put in a jar with a lid. Let sit for 24 hours and stir again. Do not make the bathwater too hot, as the oils will dissipate. Do not add the salts when the water is running, but add ½ cup of the bath salt mixture and the milk to the water as you get into the tub. Oftentimes people add 1 tablespoon milk to the water; this will cause the essential oil to blend into the water and not float on top. Store the remainder in a jar with a tight-fitting lid, in a cool, dark area, for up to 3 months.

CALM ME AIR

This diffuse recipe helped me so much when I was going through menopause. I would be extremely angry one minute and crying the next for no real reason. This helped me to remain calm and levelheaded through many bad days. This recipe contains therapeutic properties such as antidepressant, analgesic, nervine, purifying, and restorative elements.

YIELD: 1 APPLICATION

4 drops lavender oil
3 drops angelica oil

2 drops basil oil
2 drops wild orange oil
1 drop sage oil
Water

Most diffusers come with directions for using essential oils. Add the manufacturer's recommended amount of water and the oils to the diffuser and run your delightful diffuser several times a day to receive the desired effect.

COOL SHEETS POWDER

Bring those nasty night sweats under control with this cool-inducing powder. These essential oils have naturally cooling properties to bring you relief and a great night's sleep.

YIELD: 10 TO 20 APPLICATIONS

10 drops peppermint oil
8 drops orange oil
5 drops chamomile oil
½ cup cornstarch

Combine the ingredients very well with a whisk. Pour into a mason jar with holes poked into the lid. Shake the powder inside a pillowcase or under the sheets, and wake up in the morning with renewed energy after a cool, peaceful night's sleep. When storing your jar, you can place a piece of plastic wrap under the lid so that the powder won't spill out of the jar. Store in a jar with a tight-fitting lid, in a cool, dark, dry area, for up to 3 months.

MENSTRUAL CRAMPS

Menstrual cramps can range from slightly annoying to excruciatingly painful. Essential oils rubbed on the abdomen or in a bath can be useful in soothing and calming the contracting muscles and relieving the pain.

Essential Oils: chamomile, marjoram, melissa, geranium, cypress, clary sage, yarrow, fennel, rose, basil, lavender, peppermint, birch, ginger, jasmine, and rosemary

CRAMP RUB

The monthly period can often be very painful. This rub will help to alleviate cramps by using essential oils to relax muscles and end your pain. The pain-relieving properties in this rub include antispasmodic, carminative, analgesic, uterine, and anesthetic components.

YIELD: 2 TO 6 APPLICATIONS

4 drops clary sage oil

3 drops lavender oil

2 drops peppermint oil

1 drop yarrow oil

1 ounce carrier oil

In a small container, drip the essential oils. Pour in the carrier oil and swirl to mix the oils. Rub the abdomen or desired area lightly with your fingertips or a soft cloth dipped into the mixture to ensure that the essential oils are distributed over the skin. You can also pour into a roll-on bottle and roll onto the desired area. Be sure not to get any into the eyes or sensitive areas. Store unused portion in a jar with a tight-fitting lid, in a cool, dark area, for up to 3 months.

MUSCLE-RELAXING BATH

When cramping is very painful, these oils will help to reduce that pain so that you can get back to living life. The pain-reducing elements in this recipe include analgesic, antispasmodic, sedative, and anti-inflammatory properties.

Yield: 1 application

7 drops lavender oil

6 drops chamomile oil

3 drops jasmine oil

2 drops geranium oil

2 drops rose oil

1 tablespoon carrier oil

1 tablespoon milk (optional for adults, recommended for children)

While the bathwater is running, pour the ingredients into the bath. Make sure that the water is not so hot as to cause the essential oils to dissipate. Oftentimes people add 1 tablespoon milk to the water; this will cause the essential oil to blend into the water and not float on top. Soak in the water as long as you are comfortable.

I GOT YOUR BACK MASSAGE

This massage will help you get through those aches and pains. The sensual nature of the massage will relax those tense muscles and bring much-needed relief. The essential oils will relax you and make you feel like a million bucks with their analgesic, antispasmodic, and anti-inflammatory properties.

Yield: 2 to 6 applications

4 drops basil oil

3 drops rose oil

2 drops ginger oil

1 ounce carrier oil

In a small container, drip the essential oils. Pour in the carrier oil and swirl to mix the oils. Rub the abdomen, back, or desired area lightly with your fingertips or a soft cloth dipped into the mixture to ensure that the essential oils are distributed over the skin. You can also pour into a roll-on bottle and roll onto the desired area. Be sure not to get any into the eyes or sensitive areas. Store unused portion in a jar with a tight-fitting lid, in a cool, dark area, for up to 3 months.

MIGRAINE

It's unclear why some people are prone to migraines and others never have them at all. There is no known cure for migraines, but often a food allergy is at the root of this problem. The food elimination diet, which cuts out dairy, sugar, eggs, or wheat, can sometimes eliminate migraines altogether, and these essential oils can help reduce the pain. If it's chronic or severe, seek medical attention to rule out anything more serious.

Essential Oils: lavender, marjoram, peppermint, basil, eucalyptus, Roman chamomile, clary sage, neroli, valerian, angelica, ginger, frankincense, birch, rosemary, wintergreen, coriander, honeysuckle, linden blossom, spearmint, and spikenard

CALE'S RAPID CURE

My grandson has terrible migraines, and this is what helps him the most. I just dab a drop of one of these oils on his temples and before you know it he is out of his bed and playing with his brothers. The therapeutic properties in these oils include analgesic, anti-inflammatory, and antispasmodic agents.

YIELD: 1 APPLICATION

1 drop lavender oil, or 1 drop myrrh oil, or 1 drop peppermint oil

A few essential oils can be placed directly on the skin (neat) without adding carrier oil to them. Ensure that you are using a safe, pure-grade essential oil before placing on the body, as essential oils can be very powerful. Apply one drop to the temples, forehead, or back of the neck, and relax in a cool, dark area until you can bear humanity again.

MIGRAINE COMPRESS

This compress can work wonders while you lay down and rest. Wake up after using a compress with these essential oils in it and be migraine free! This blend contains analgesic, anesthetic, antispasmodic, and vasoconstrictor therapeutic properties to bring comfort and stop the pain.

YIELD: 1 APPLICATION

1 drop frankincense oil
1 drop peppermint oil
1 drop basil oil
1 drop lavender oil
1 wet cloth

Use gauze, linen, or any comfortable, clean damp cloth. With an eye dropper, drop oils onto the cloth and place over the temple area, back of the neck, or forehead. Leave the cloth on until it is no longer cool, 15 to 30 minutes.

MIGRAINE HAND SOAK

It does seem strange that soaking your hand could relieve such massive pain in your head, but it's true! Give this hand soak a try with its analgesic, antispasmodic, and anti-inflammatory properties.

YIELD: 1 APPLICATION

4 drops lavender oil
4 drops ginger oil
2 cups hot water

Mix the ingredients in a bowl. Make sure the water is not too hot, and soak your hands alternately until you find relief. Use the solution throughout day and discard the remainder at day's end.

MOTION SICKNESS

Some people get motion sickness in the car, others on boats or planes. It's very unpleasant and can sometimes cause severe vomiting and stomach cramps. Essential oils can alleviate these symptoms or even rid your body of motion sickness altogether.

Essential Oils: peppermint, ginger, fennel, chamomile, dill, thyme, rosemary, myrrh, marjoram, lemongrass, basil, cinnamon, lavender, grapefruit, frankincense, and eucalyptus

QUEASY RUB

My family, to dispel the awful feelings associated with motion sickness, has used these essential oils for a long time with great success. These essential oils contain analgesic, antigalactogogue, antispasmodic, digestive, and stomachic properties.

YIELD: 4 TO 10 APPLICATIONS

4 drops peppermint oil
3 drops chamomile oil
2 drops dill oil
2 drops myrrh oil
2 ounces carrier oil

In a small container, drip the essential oils. Pour in the carrier oil and swirl to mix the oils. Rub the desired area lightly with your fingertips or a soft cloth dipped into the mixture to ensure that the essential oils are distributed over the skin. You can also pour into a roll-on bottle and roll onto the desired area. Be sure not to get any into the eyes or sensitive areas. Store the remainder in a jar with a tight-fitting lid, in a cool, dark area, for up to 3 months.

TUMMY RUB

Use this rub to quell nausea and feel great again. The elements in this recipe include antiemetic, anti-inflammatory, and antispasmodic properties, to name a few. Take this on your next cruise and you will be able to dance and party with the best of them!

YIELD: 2 TO 6 APPLICATIONS

2 drops lemongrass oil
2 drops fennel oil
2 drops chamomile oil
1 ounce carrier oil

In a small container, drip the essential oils. Pour in the carrier oil and swirl to mix the oils. Rub the chest, stomach, forehead, neck, or desired area lightly with your fingertips or a soft cloth dipped into the mixture to ensure that the es-

sential oils are distributed over the skin. You can also pour into a roll-on bottle and roll onto the desired area. Be sure not to get any into the eyes or sensitive areas. Store unused portion in a jar with a tight-fitting lid, in a cool, dark area, for up to 3 months.

NAUSEA INHALE

It's easy to carry a small vial of essential oil with you so that you can put a halt to those bad effects of motion sickness. The nausea-fighting elements in these oils are analgesic, antiemetic, and antispasmodic properties.

YIELD: 1 APPLICATION

1 drop peppermint oil, or 1 drop lavender oil, or 1 drop ginger oil

Place the drop of essential oil on a handkerchief or tissue, in the palm of your hand, or in an essential oil inhaler. Cup to your nose and inhale the aroma. Repeat several times daily or as needed.

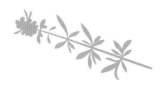

MUSCLE/ LIGAMENT/ TENDON PAIN

There are so many reasons you might have pain in your muscles, ligaments, or tendons. Overwork, too much exercise, illness, inactivity—the list is endless. After receiving medical attention and ruling out any tears to the body, or other more serious causes of the pain, essential oils can be used to reduce swelling and pain and to speed healing.

Essential Oils: arnica, basil, lavender, chamomile, ginger, marjoram, rosemary, camphor, birch, eucalyptus, thyme, black pepper, vetiver, lemongrass, jasmine, melissa, lemon, wintergreen, sage, pine, peppermint, niaouli, juniper, helichrysum, frankincense, oregano, cajeput, and clary sage

MUSCLE PAIN BATH SALTS

When those aches and pains get to be too much, the salts and the essential oils in this bath will have you feeling like you can tackle anything. A few of the muscle-relieving elements in this recipe have analgesic, antispasmodic, and anti-

rheumatic therapeutic properties.

YIELD: 5 TO 6 APPLICATIONS

7 drops cajeput essential oil
7 drops vetiver oil
7 drops niaouli oil
2 tablespoons carrier oil
3 cups salts (pink Himalayan salt, sea salt, or Epsom salts)
1 tablespoon milk (optional for adults, recommended for children)

Add the oils to the salt. Stir until the mixture is well blended. Put in a jar with a lid. Let sit for 24 hours and stir again. Do not make the bathwater too hot, as the oils will dissipate. Do not add the salts when the water is running, but add ½ cup of the bath salt mixture and the milk to the water as you get into the tub. Oftentimes people add 1 tablespoon milk to the water; this will cause the essential oil to blend into the water and not float on top. Store the remainder in a jar with a tight-fitting lid, in a cool, dark area, for up to 3 months.

MUSCLE RUB

The healing benefits of this rub are quick and deep. Use this when you have a particular muscle or ligament giving you problems. The therapeutic properties at work in this blend include analgesic, antispasmodic, anti-inflammatory, and antirheumatic elements.

YIELD: 4 TO 10 APPLICATIONS

12 drops lavender oil
5 drops marjoram oil
3 drops chamomile oil
3 drops ginger oil
2 ounces carrier oil

In a small container, drip the essential oils. Pour in the carrier oil and swirl to mix the oils. Rub the sore muscle area lightly with your fingertips or a soft cloth dipped into the mixture to ensure that the essential oils are distributed over the skin. You can also pour into a roll-on bottle and roll onto the desired area. Be sure not to get any into the eyes or sensitive areas. Store unused portion in a jar with a tight fitting lid, in a cool, dark area for up to one month.

LEVI'S MUSCLE COMPRESS

When lifting weights or too much exercise make your muscles hurt the next day, apply this compress of essential oils and you will feel better in no time. The therapeutic properties that bring quick relief include antirheumatic, analgesic, anti-inflammatory, and antispasmodic agents.

YIELD: 1 APPLICATION

6 drops niaouli oil

4 drops vetiver oil
3 drops rosemary oil
1 damp cloth

Use gauze, linen, or any comfortable, clean, damp cloth. Mix the ingredients, pour onto the cloth, and place over the sore muscles or the affected area. This is a great recipe for after a workout or lifting weights.

MUSCLE SPASM

An involuntary, often painful, and usually repeated contraction in a muscle or a group of muscles. Essential oils can bring relief to someone with severe muscle spasms, and a physician can diagnose whether you are in need of more serious assistance, such as surgery or rehabilitation exercises.

Essential Oils: marjoram, Roman chamomile, basil, cypress, lime, geranium, helichrysum, black pepper, rosemary, vetiver, petitgrain, clary sage, fennel, arnica, and frankincense

HEAL ME NOW RUB

The essential oils in this rub are wonderful for

ending muscle spasm pain and the cramping aches that follow. The agents at work in this blend include antispasmodic, euphoric, nervine, analgesic, and anti-inflammatory properties.

YIELD: 4 TO 10 APPLICATIONS

5 drops marjoram oil

4 drops Roman chamomile oil

3 drops clary sage oil

3 drops arnica oil

1 drop black pepper oil

2 ounces carrier oil

In a small container, drip the essential oils. Pour in the carrier oil and swirl to mix the oils. Rub the muscles or desired area lightly with your fingertips or a soft cloth dipped into the mixture to ensure that the essential oils are distributed over the skin. You can also pour into a roll-on bottle and roll onto the desired area. Be sure not to get any into the eyes or sensitive areas. Store unused portion in a jar with a tight fitting lid, in a cool, dark area for up to one month.

HEATH'S POULTICE

This is the perfect poultice for healing aching muscles after a strenuous workout. The therapeutic properties in this blend include analgesic, anti-inflammatory, antispasmodic, and restorative elements.

YIELD: 1 APPLICATION

3 drops basil oil

3 drops lavender oil

2 drops vetiver oil

1 ounce carrier oil

1 damp cloth

Mix the ingredients and apply them with a dropper to a clean, damp, warm cloth and place on the affected area. When the poultice gets too cool or dry, reapply as needed. Store any of the remaining mixture in a jar with a tight-fitting lid, in a cool, dark area, for up to 3 months.

JACKIE'S SILKY SOAK

This heavenly feeling recipe will bring comfort and healing to those tired, sore, and achy muscles. Take this bath at night, as the soothing properties will have you wanting to crawl into your bed and sleep all night. The healing elements of this blend include antispasmodic, sedative, anti-inflammatory, and analgesic properties.

YIELD: 1 APPLICATION

4 drops petitgrain oil

4 drops cypress oil

3 drops geranium oil

2 drops rosemary oil

1 tablespoon milk (optional for adults, recommended for children)

As the bathwater is running, pour the oils into the bath. Make sure that the water is not so hot as to cause the essential oils to dissipate. Oftentimes people add 1 tablespoon milk to the water; this will cause the essential oil to blend into the water and not float on top. Soak in the water as long as your are comfortable.

VANCE'S MUSCLE-HEALING MASSAGE

Not only will the massage help to alleviate your muscle pain, but also the essential oils in this recipe work like magic to heal and repair muscle spasms with their analgesic, anti-inflammatory, antispasmodic, and restorative properties.

YIELD: 4 TO 10 APPLICATIONS

3 drops basil oil
3 drops marjoram oil
3 drops lavender oil
3 drops Roman chamomile oil
3 drops rosemary oil
2 ounces carrier oil

In a small container, drip the essential oils. Pour in the carrier oil and swirl to mix the oils. Rub the sore muscles lightly with your fingertips or a soft cloth dipped into the mixture to ensure that the essential oils are distributed over the skin. You can also pour into a roll-on bottle and roll onto the desired area. Be sure not to get any into the eyes or sensitive areas. Store the remainder in a jar with a tight-fitting lid, in a cool, dark area, for up to 3 months.

NAUSEA

There are many reasons for nausea: pregnancy, motion sickness, dizziness, emotions, vertigo, and hundreds of illnesses, both mild and/or chronic. Essential oils are famous for helping to reduce nausea in many individuals. Be sure to read the warnings in this book in the event you may be pregnant. Many essential oils are extremely dangerous for pregnant women.

Essential Oils: peppermint, fennel, Roman chamomile, ginger, basil, spearmint, cardamom oil, lemongrass, bergamot, coriander, dill, patchouli, sandalwood, rose, black pepper, melissa, clove, cinnamon, eucalyptus, frankincense, grapefruit, marjoram, myrrh, rosemary, and thyme

TUMMY OIL

People have chewed on fennel seeds for thousands of years to alleviate nausea. Now we don't have to chew the bitter seed, we can just rub on this blend of essential oils to get that nauseated feeling to disappear. The tummy trouble–fighting elements of this blend include antiinflammatory, antiemetic, and antispasmodic properties.

YIELD: 2 TO 4 APPLICATIONS

3 drops lemongrass oil
2 drops chamomile oil
1 drop fennel oil
1 ounce carrier oil

In a small container, drip the essential oils. Pour in the carrier oil and swirl to mix the oils. Rub the stomach and chest area lightly with your fingertips or a soft cloth dipped into the mixture to ensure that the essential oils are distributed over the skin. You can also pour into a roll-on bottle and roll onto the desired area. Be sure not to get any into the eyes or sensitive areas. Repeat throughout the day as needed. Store the remainder in a jar with a tight-fitting lid, in a cool, dark area, for up to 3 months.

NAUSEA-REDUCING DIFFUSER

While some smells cause us to get nauseated, other smells can cause nausea to stop! These essential oils are packed full of tummy-soothing,

healing properties such as analgesic, antispasmodic, and digestive agents.

YIELD: 1 APPLICATION

4 drops lavender oil
4 drops bergamot oil
Water

Most diffusers come with directions for using essential oils. Add the manufacturer's recommended amount of water and the oils to the diffuser and run your delightful diffuser several times a day to receive the desired effect.

INSTANT RELIEF

It has long been known that just smelling peppermint oil can stop a person from feeling sick. Carry this with you in a small vial to use as needed. The nausea-reducing therapeutic properties of peppermint oil are anti-inflammatory, digestive, nervine, stomachic, and anesthetic.

YIELD: 1 APPLICATION

2 drops peppermint oil

Place the drops of essential oil on a handkerchief or tissue, in the palm of your hand, or in an essential oil inhaler. Cup to your nose and inhale the aroma. Repeat several times daily or as needed.

TUMMY RUB

This is an age-old essential oil recipe that has been used in my family for many years. The stomachache-healing properties in this blend are anti-inflammatory, antiemetic, antiseptic, digestive, and antispasmodic.

YIELD: 2 TO 6 APPLICATIONS

3 drops peppermint oil
2 drops basil oil
2 drops fennel oil
1 ounce carrier oil

In a small container, drip the essential oils. Pour in the carrier oil and swirl to mix the oils. Rub the stomach area lightly with your fingertips or a soft cloth dipped into the mixture to ensure that the essential oils are distributed over the skin. You can also pour into a roll-on bottle and roll onto the desired area. Be sure not to get any into the eyes or sensitive areas. Store unused portion in a jar with a tight-fitting lid, in a cool, dark area, for up to 3 months.

TUMMY ACHE DRINK

Peppermint essential oil is one of the quickest ways to get you feeling better quickly. The peppermint contains analgesic, anti-inflammatory, antispasmodic, cordial, digestive, and stomachic properties.

YIELD: 1 TO 2 APPLICATIONS

1 drop peppermint oil
2 ounces water

Ensure that your essential oil is safe for consumption and internal use and is clinical/therapeutic grade. Mix the oil and water and drink slowly. Store unused portion in a jar with a tight-fitting lid, in a cool, dark area or the refrigerator, for up to 1 day.

TUMMY COMPRESS

My family has used these three essential oils, successfully, for years. The healing components in this blend include antispasmodic, carminative, digestive, stomachic, and sudorific elements.

YIELD: 1 APPLICATION

2 drops ginger oil
1 drop dill oil
1 drop frankincense oil
1 tablespoon carrier oil

Mix the ingredients together in a small container. Dip a soft cloth into the mixture and lay the cloth on the stomach for 15 to 30 minutes. Repeat as needed.

NECK PAIN

Neck pain can range from annoying to very serious. There is so much activity in the neck area, from the spinal cord to the vocal cords. Essential oils can help in reducing milder neck pain, from a crick in the neck to muscle strain. Ensure that a physician diagnoses the problem if pain persists.

Essential Oils: birch, frankincense, helichrysum, lavender, rosemary, peppermint, oregano, myrrh, white fir, wintergreen, basil, cypress, eucalyptus, thyme, lemon, lime, marjoram, and vetiver

TURN THAT HEAD POULTICE

The plants and herbs that these essential oils are derived from have long been used for those times when we sleep wrong and get a "crick" in our neck. These essential oils will have you loosened up and ready to drive in no time. The healing elements in this blend include analgesic, anti-inflammatory, antispasmodic, and anesthetic properties.

YIELD: 1 APPLICATION

2 drops lemon oil
1 drop thyme oil
1 drop lavender oil
1 drop peppermint oil
1 wet cloth

Drip the essential oils onto a clean, damp, warm cloth with an eye dropper and place on the neck in the affected area. When the poultice gets too cool or dry, add water and reapply as needed.

NATURAL MUSCLE-RELAXING SOAK

This recipe contains essential oils that calm and relax your mind and all of your muscles with their analgesic, antispasmodic, nervine, sedative, and vasodilator properties.

YIELD: 1 APPLICATION

5 drops lavender oil
4 drops vetiver oil
3 drops marjoram oil
1 tablespoon carrier oil
1 tablespoon milk (optional for adults, recommended for children)

While the bathwater is running, pour the ingredients into the bath. Make sure that the water is not so hot as to cause the essential oils to dissipate. Oftentimes people add 1 tablespoon milk to the water; this will cause the essential oils to blend into the water and not float on top. Make sure the neck is resting in the water on a bath pillow. Soak your bath cloth in the water and re-apply often to your neck area. Soak in the water as long as you are comfortable.

CHEMICAL-FREE RUB

Carry this little magic recipe with you to apply when the stiffness sets in and you are in need of something to help you keep going but you don't want to take any pain pills. The natural healing properties of this recipe include analgesic, antispasmodic, anti-inflammatory, and restorative elements.

YIELD: 2 TO 6 APPLICATIONS

3 drops vetiver oil
2 drops lime oil
2 drops myrrh oil
1 ounce carrier oil

In a small container, drip the essential oils. Pour in the carrier oil and swirl to mix the oils. Rub the back of the neck area lightly with your fingertips or a soft cloth dipped into the mixture to ensure that the essential oils are distributed over the skin. You can also pour into a roll-on bottle and roll onto the desired area. Be sure not to get any into the eyes or sensitive areas. Store unused portion in a jar with a tight-fitting lid, in a cool, dark area, for up to 3 months.

NERVE PAIN
(Neuralgia)

There are various causes for nerve pain: sciatica, diabetes, nerve damage, and a host of illnesses. It can be debilitating and painful. The plants from which we derive our essential oils have been used for centuries to reduce nerve pain in individuals. Always consult a physician to rule out serious causes.

Essential Oils: helichrysum, lavender, Roman chamomile, black pepper, peppermint, marjoram, ginger, oregano, lemongrass, lemon, grapefruit, cassia, birch, rosemary, pine, eucalyptus, juniper, vetiver, cypress, clove, sandalwood, and patchouli

DADDY TOM'S LEG RUB

This is a rub that works well on my dad's painful legs. Just rub it in and let the essential oils do their job. The healing components in this blend include therapeutic properties such as anti-inflammatory, antispasmodic, anticoagulant, analgesic, antineuralgic, and antivenous agents.

YIELD: 4 TO 10 APPLICATIONS

5 drops chamomile oil

3 drops marjoram oil

3 drops helichrysum oil

2 drops lavender oil

2 ounces carrier oil

In a small container, drip the essential oils. Pour in the carrier oil and swirl to mix the oils. Rub the legs lightly with your fingertips or a soft cloth dipped into the mixture to ensure that the essential oils are distributed over the skin. You can also pour into a roll-on bottle and roll onto the desired area. Be sure not to get any into the eyes or sensitive areas. Store the remainder in a jar with a tight-fitting lid, in a cool, dark area, for up to 3 months.

SHARP PAIN MASSAGE

This blend will provide instant relief that lasts for hours. These essential oils work together to calm the nerve pain and relax the patient with their analgesic, anti-inflammatory, sedative, antineuralgic, and antispasmodic properties.

YIELD: 2 TO 6 APPLICATIONS

3 drops chamomile oil

3 drops black pepper oil

3 drops lavender oil

1 drop clove oil

1 ounce carrier oil

In a small container, drip the essential oils. Pour in the carrier oil and swirl to mix the oils. Rub the area of nerve pain lightly with your fingertips or a soft cloth dipped into the mixture to ensure that the essential oils are distributed over the skin. You can also pour into a roll-on bottle and roll onto the desired area. Be sure not to get any into the eyes or sensitive areas. Store unused portion in a jar with a tight-fitting lid, in a cool, dark area, for up to 3 months.

BATHE ME INTO TRANQUILITY

These relaxing essential oils will have you zoned out and pain free in minutes. The agents at work here include analgesic, antispasmodic, anti-inflammatory, and nervine properties.

YIELD: 1 APPLICATION

6 drops lavender oil

4 drops eucalyptus oil

4 drops patchouli oil

1 tablespoon carrier oil

1 tablespoon milk (optional for adults, recommended for children)

While the bathwater is running, pour the ingredients into the bath. Make sure that the water is not so hot as to cause the essential oils to dissipate. Oftentimes people add 1 tablespoon milk to the water; this will cause the essential oil to blend into the water and not float on top. Soak in the water as long as you are comfortable.

NOSEBLEED

A nosebleed can happen for any reason—or sometimes for apparently no reason at all! Children often have nosebleeds that dissipate after a few minutes. If a person continues to bleed heavily after several minutes, a trip to the ER may be in order so that a physician can evaluate the situation.

Essential Oils: lavender, lemon, cypress, frankincense, and helichrysum

SMELL IT AWAY

This is an old trick that works well and causes no stress, with its hemostatic properties.

YIELD: 1 APPLICATION

1 drop lemon oil, or 1 drop lavender oil

Place the drop of essential oil on a handkerchief or tissue, in the palm of your hand, or in an essential oil inhaler. Cup to your nose and inhale the aroma. Repeat several times daily or as needed.

CALE'S BLOODY RUB

This recipe can be applied outside of the nose; when the essential oils are inhaled, the bleeding slowly comes to a halt due to the hemostatic properties.

YIELD: 1 APPLICATION

1 drop lemon oil
1 drop lavender oil
1 drop cypress oil
½ teaspoon carrier oil

In a small container, drip the essential oils. Pour in the carrier oil and swirl to mix the oils. Rub the outer nostril area lightly with your fingertips or a soft cloth dipped into the mixture to ensure that the essential oils are distributed over the skin. You can also pour into a roll-on bottle and roll onto the desired area. Be sure not to get any into the eyes or sensitive areas. If any of the mixture remains, store in a container with a tight-fitting lid in the refrigerator for up to 3 days.

OBESITY

Oftentimes a person is overweight due to emotional issues, hereditary factors, food addiction, and inactivity. Obesity can lead to many serious medical consequences. Essential oils can help give you more energy to move around, or to feel more peaceful, thereby redirecting emotional eating, and to feel better about yourself.

Essential Oils: grapefruit, lemon, peppermint, cypress, lavender, fennel, cinnamon, ginger, dill, patchouli, oregano, mandarin, juniper, white birch, lime, basil, rosemary, eucalyptus, ylang-ylang, and orange

ENERGIZING BATH SALTS

These essential oils will energize you to the point that you are ready to give that workout a shot. Go for it! These energizing essential oils contain restorative, tonic, and stimulant agents.

Yield: 5 to 6 applications

7 drops lime oil
7 drops ylang-ylang oil
7 drops grapefruit oil
2 tablespoons carrier oil
3 cups salts (pink Himalayan salt, sea salt, or Epsom salts)

1 tablespoon milk (optional for adults, recommended for children)

Add the oils to the salt. Stir until the mixture is well blended. Put in a jar with a lid. Let sit for 24 hours and stir again. Do not make the bathwater too hot, as the oils will dissipate. Do not add the salts when the water is running, but add ½ cup of the bath salt mixture and the milk to the water as you get into the tub. Oftentimes people add 1 tablespoon milk to the water; this will cause the essential oil to blend into the water and not float on top. Store the remainder in a jar with a tight-fitting lid, in a cool, dark area, for up to 3 months.

RUB IT AWAY

It has long been reported that grapefruit oil has the ability to rid the body of cellulite. This is a recipe for those who wish to give it a try with its lymphatic, stimulant, diuretic, and tonic properties.

Yield: 4 to 10 applications

2 drops grapefruit oil
2 drops peppermint oil
2 drops cypress oil
2 drops lavender oil
2 ounces carrier oil

In a small container, drip the essential oils. Pour

in the carrier oil and swirl to mix the oils. Rub the desired area lightly with your fingertips or a soft cloth dipped into the mixture to ensure that the essential oils are distributed over the skin. You can also pour into a roll-on bottle and roll onto the desired area. Be sure not to get any into the eyes or sensitive areas. Store the remainder in a jar with a tight-fitting lid, in a cool, dark area, for up to 3 months.

SKINNY BATH TONIC

This bath recipe includes essential oils that may assist in weight loss, increase energy, and make you and your home smell great! The oils in this bath include tonic, diuretic, antitoxic, and stomachic properties.

YIELD: 1 APPLICATION

5 drops grapefruit oil
4 drops juniper oil
3 drops orange oil
1 tablespoon carrier oil
1 tablespoon milk (optional for adults, recommended for children)

While the bathwater is running, pour the ingredients into the bath. Make sure that the water is not so hot as to cause the essential oils to dissipate. Oftentimes people add 1 tablespoon milk to the water; this will cause the essential oil to blend into the water and not float on top. Soak in the water as long as you are comfortable.

OCD
(Obsessive-Compulsive Disorder)

Locking and unlocking doors, washing the hands repeatedly, obsessively organizing things, and counting and repeating words can be symptoms of OCD. Therapy and new medications offer hope to many who suffer from chronic OCD and are available from medical professionals. Essential oils can be used to bring calmness to a situation where someone suffering from OCD could have an issue. OCD runs in my family, materializing as "tics" or obsessively collecting items (hoarding). These essential oils have brought much relief in times of overwhelming stress and OCD overload.

Essential Oils: lavender, sandalwood, vetiver, bergamot, ylang-ylang, patchouli, geranium, frankincense, and cypress

I AM UNIQUE

Just run this little recipe in your diffuser and feel the calm invade the air with its antidepressant and sedative properties.

YIELD: 1 APPLICATION

3 drops patchouli oil
3 drops bergamot oil
2 drops lavender oil
Water

Most diffusers come with directions for using essential oils. Add the manufacturer's recommended amount of water and the oils to the diffuser and run your delightful diffuser several times a day to receive the desired effect.

STOP THE PATTERN BATH

If you can remove the person from the stressful situation and let them take this calming, peaceful bath, just watch as their mood changes from frantic to blissful. The calming essential oils in this recipe contain sedative, tranquilizing, and antidepressant properties.

YIELD: 1 APPLICATION

5 drops cypress oil
5 drops vetiver oil
5 drops lavender oil
1 tablespoon carrier oil

1 tablespoon milk (optional for adults, recommended for children)

While the bathwater is running, pour the ingredients into the bath. Make sure that the water is not so hot as to cause the essential oils to dissipate. Oftentimes people add 1 tablespoon milk to the water; this will cause the essential oils to blend into the water and not float on top. Soak in the water as long as you are comfortable.

REPEATER INHALER

This is a quick fix that can be carried in your purse and used in emergencies, such as in a crowded department store! The properties in these oils contain antidepressant, sedative, and calming agents.

YIELD: 1 APPLICATION

1 drop lavender oil, or 1 drop frankincense oil

Place the drop of essential oil on a handkerchief or tissue, in the palm of your hand, or in an essential oil inhaler. Cup to your nose and inhale the aroma. Repeat several times daily or as needed.

OSTEOARTHRITIS

New medications offer relief and remission for many sufferers of this degenerative arthritis affecting the cartilage and the joints. Lifestyle changes, diet, and exercise can be extremely helpful in controlling the severity of this disease. Essential oils can assist with many aspects of osteoarthritis such as pain, stress relief, and energy for exercise. Be sure to check with your doctor to ensure that the essential oils won't interfere with your medications.

Essential Oils: birch, frankincense, lavender, sandalwood, lime, ginger, German chamomile, wintergreen, lemon, marjoram, myrrh, oregano, peppermint, eucalyptus, and geranium

PLEASING RUB

Rub this blend on your aching joints and bones and get quick, pleasing relief from its analgesic, anti-inflammatory, and antispasmodic properties.

YIELD: 4 TO 10 APPLICATIONS

4 drops myrrh oil
3 drops lemongrass oil
2 drops vetiver oil
2 drops eucalyptus oil
2 ounces carrier oil

In a small container, drip the essential oils. Pour in the carrier oil and swirl to mix the oils. Rub the desired area lightly with your fingertips or a soft cloth dipped into the mixture to ensure that the essential oils are distributed over the skin. You can also pour into a roll-on bottle and roll onto the desired area. Be sure not to get any into the eyes or sensitive areas. Store the remainder in a jar with a tight-fitting lid, in a cool, dark area, for up to 3 months.

IT'S GONNA SNOW MASSAGE OIL

This is a good "weather changing" rub that I use on myself when those aches are so sharp and painful. The essential oils in this blend contain analgesic, anesthetic, anti-inflammatory, nervine, anesthetic, and vasoconstrictor elements.

YIELD: 4 TO 10 APPLICATIONS

4 drops frankincense oil
2 drops lemon oil
2 drops peppermint oil
2 drops vetiver oil
2 ounces carrier oil

In a small container, drip the essential oils. Pour in the carrier oil and swirl to mix the oils. Rub the painful joint and muscle areas lightly with your fingertips or a soft cloth dipped into the mixture to ensure that the essential oils are distributed over the skin. You can also pour into a roll-on bottle and roll onto the desired area. Be sure not to get any into the eyes or sensitive areas. This can be reapplied as often as needed. Store the remainder in a jar with a tight-fitting lid, in a cool, dark area, for up to 3 months.

RELIEVING BATH

These healing essential oils will bring much-needed relief to your aching bones and muscles with their analgesic, anti-inflammatory, antirheumatic, and antispasmodic therapeutic properties.

YIELD: 1 APPLICATION

5 drops lavender oil
3 drops geranium oil
3 drops frankincense oil
2 drops German chamomile oil
1 tablespoon carrier oil
1 tablespoon milk (optional for adults, recommended for children)

While the bathwater is running, pour the ingredients into the bath. Make sure that the water is not so hot as to cause the essential oils to dissipate. Oftentimes people add 1 tablespoon milk to the water; this will cause the essential oils to blend into the water and not float on top. Soak in the water as long as you are comfortable.

PANIC ATTACKS

A panic attack often feels like a heart attack. Your heart rate elevates, your throat muscles constrict, your thoughts race, and the "fight or flight" chemicals course through your body. If you do think you're having a heart attack, you must seek medical help. Once anything more serious has been ruled out, try these recipes to supplement any other methods you're using to manage your stress. Essential oils can help calm you down, which is the number one goal during a panic attack.

Essential Oils Used: lavender, frankincense, rosemary, linden blossom, and ylang-ylang

CALM ME DOWN AIR

This is a calming diffuser that contains essential oils that will help a person to remain calm and clearheaded. The components of this blend contain antidepressant, anti-inflammatory, detoxifying, restorative, and sedative elements.

YIELD: 1 APPLICATION

3 drops lemon oil
3 drops lavender oil
3 drops linden blossom oil
Water

Most diffusers come with directions for using essential oils. Add the manufacturer's recommended amount of water and the oils to the diffuser and run your delightful diffuser several times a day to receive the desired effect.

BREATHE DEEPLY POULTICE

This is a great way to end a panic attack if it is in progress. Just place on the back of the neck and tell the person to breathe deeply. They will come out the other side of the attack in minutes. The responsible agents in this recipe are sedative and antidepressant, and relieve irritability and nervous tension.

YIELD: 1 APPLICATION

2 drops frankincense oil
2 drops lavender oil
2 drops ylang-ylang oil
1 wet cloth

Apply the oils to a clean, damp, warm cloth with an eye dropper and place on the back of the neck or head. When the poultice gets too cool or dry, reapply as needed.

ONE CONSCIOUSNESS BATH

These essential oils will silence your scattered, troubling thoughts and help you to focus. The components of this blend contain antidepres-sant, restorative, sedative, and tonic therapeutic properties.

YIELD: 1 APPLICATION

4 drops lavender oil
4 drops frankincense oil
4 drops linden blossom oil
1 tablespoon carrier oil
*1 tablespoon milk (optional for adults,
    recommended for children)*

While the bathwater is running, pour the ingredients into the bath. Make sure that the water is not so hot as to cause the essential oils to dissipate. Oftentimes people add 1 tablespoon milk to the water; this will cause the essential oil to blend into the water and not float on top. Soak in the water as long as you are comfortable.

I'LL BE FINE MASSAGE

Using these particular oils in a massage is a surefire way to calm and relax a person. This blend contains restorative, tonic, and antidepressant elements.

YIELD: 2 TO 6 APPLICATIONS

3 drops lavender oil
3 drops frankincense oil
2 drops rosemary oil
1 ounce carrier oil

In a small container, drip the essential oils. Pour in the carrier oil and swirl to mix the oils. Rub the desired area lightly with your fingertips or a soft cloth dipped into the mixture to ensure that the essential oils are distributed over the skin. You can also pour into a roll-on bottle and roll onto the desired area. Be sure not to get any into the eyes or sensitive areas. Store unused portion in a jar with a tight-fitting lid, in a cool, dark area, for up to 3 months.

PERIODONTAL DISEASE

Gum disease can lead to tooth loss when the bone and gums become so infected that they can no longer hold the teeth in place. Dental treatments can often curb this disease, and the outlook is great when caught early. Oil pulling can be very effective in ending periodontal disease and protecting the teeth and gums. Be sure to talk to your dentist before starting an essential oil regimen for your gums.

Essential Oils: tea tree (melaleuca), myrrh, clove, lavender, lemon, fennel, manuka, oregano, rosemary, frankincense, helichrysum, and eucalyptus

TOOTH PAIN ENDER

I used this when my toothache caused by periodontal disease had the whole side of my head and my ear hurting. It brought instantaneous relief with its analgesic, anti-inflammatory, antimicrobial, and antiseptic properties.

Yield: 1 application

1 drop clove oil

Ensure that your essential oil is safe for consumption and internal use and is clinical/therapeutic grade. Place the drop of essential oil on a cotton ball and hold it onto the toothache. Try not to touch the oil with your tongue, as it does not taste good at all.

ESSENTIAL OIL PULL

Oil pulling is a very popular way to get the benefits of essential oils quickly and easily. This remedy is reportedly great for toothaches due to its anesthetic, analgesic, anti-infectious, anti-inflammatory, and antiseptic properties.

Yield: 1 application

3 drops myrrh oil
1 drop peppermint oil
1 tablespoon carrier oil

Ensure that your essential oil is safe for consumption and internal use and is clinical/therapeutic grade. Mix the ingredients well and swish through the teeth and mouth for 5 minutes, then spit out. Do not swallow.

MIKE'S TOOTHACHE PULL

This oil pull is full of beneficial and pain-dulling essential oils. These oils contain antibacterial, antibiotic, anti-infectious, anti-inflammatory, antimicrobial, antiseptic, antiviral, and sudorific properties.

YIELD: 1 APPLICATION

1 drop lavender oil
1 drop tea tree (melaleuca) oil
1 drop peppermint oil
1 tablespoon carrier oil

Ensure that your essential oil is safe for consumption and internal use and is clinical/therapeutic grade. Mix the ingredients in a small cup with an eye dropper or pour spout and swish through the teeth and mouth for 5 minutes, then spit out. Do not swallow.

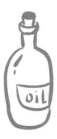

PINCHED NERVE

I've suffered pinched nerves in the past simply from reaching too far while in an awkward position. Essential oil rubs, massages, and baths can alleviate some of the pain. Medical and chiropractic care can often locate the root of the problem. Ensure through your doctor that any medications you may be on will not react negatively with the essential oils.

Essential Oils: helichrysum, sandalwood, peppermint, lavender, chamomile, and marjoram

TOMMY'S RUB

The essential oils in this rub have the healing properties needed to help end that pinching pain. The healing properties in this blend contain analgesic, anti-inflammatory, antineuralgic, and sedative elements.

YIELD: 2 TO 6 APPLICATIONS

4 drops chamomile oil
3 drops marjoram oil
3 drops helichrysum oil
2 drops lavender oil
1 ounce carrier oil

In a small container, drip the essential oils. Pour

in the carrier oil and swirl to mix the oils. Rub the desired area lightly with your fingertips or a soft cloth dipped into the mixture to ensure that the essential oils are distributed over the skin. You can also pour into a roll-on bottle and roll onto the desired area. Be sure not to get any into the eyes or sensitive areas. Store unused portion in a jar with a tight-fitting lid, in a cool, dark area, for up to 3 months.

TINA'S NERVE MASSAGE

The combination of the massage and the essential oils together work fast to bring relief to your painful condition. This blend contains anti-inflammatory, antispasmodic, and anesthetic properties.

YIELD: 4 TO 10 APPLICATIONS

5 drops sandalwood oil
5 drops peppermint oil
4 drops helichrysum oil
2 ounces carrier oil

In a small container, drip the essential oils. Pour in the carrier oil and swirl to mix the oils. Rub the desired area lightly with your fingertips or a soft cloth dipped into the mixture to ensure that the essential oils are distributed over the skin. You can also pour into a roll-on bottle and roll onto the desired area. Be sure not to get any into

the eyes or sensitive areas. Store the remainder in a jar with a tight-fitting lid, in a cool, dark area, for up to 3 months.

DANA'S PAIN-RELEASE BATH

Relax into bliss when using these essential oils in the bath. The pain-relieving properties include analgesic, anti-inflammatory, antispasmodic, and antineuralgic therapeutic elements to bring instant relief.

YIELD: 1 APPLICATION

6 drops lavender oil
4 drops chamomile oil
2 drops helichrysum oil
1 tablespoon carrier oil
1 tablespoon milk (optional for adults,
    recommended for children)

While the bathwater is running, pour the ingredients into the bath. Make sure that the water is not so hot as to cause the essential oils to dissipate. Oftentimes people add 1 tablespoon milk to the water; this will cause the essential oils to blend into the water and not float on top of the water. Soak in the water as long as you are comfortable.

PLANTER FASCIITIS

Heel pain is suffered by much of the population at some time in their lives, and it's often associated with obesity or athletics. Essential oil rubs and massages can help you overcome the pain and heal your heel!

Essential Oils: basil, wintergreen, birch, cypress, helichrysum, frankincense, myrrh, lavender, peppermint, and lemongrass

PLEASURE FOOT RUB

This healing blend combined with the foot rub will have your heel feeling much better. This combination contains antioxidant, sedative, anti-inflammatory, and nervine properties.

Yield: 1 application

1 drop helichrysum oil
1 drop lemongrass oil
1 teaspoon carrier oil

Mix the ingredients together in a small bowl. Apply the oil to the soles of the feet with your fingertips or a cotton ball and rub as often as needed. If any of the mixture remains, store in a container with a tight-fitting lid in the refrigerator for up to 3 days.

SPRING COMPRESS

Wrap this compress around your heel for fast relief and to increase your chances of getting back on your feet. This blend contains healing properties that are analgesic, anesthetic, anti-inflammatory, and sedative.

Yield: 1 application

1 drop peppermint oil
1 drop frankincense oil
1 drop basil oil
1 wet cloth

Use gauze, linen, or any soft, clean, damp cloth. Mix the oils and place them on the cloth with an eye dropper. Place the cloth over the heel or the affected area. Leave on for 15 to 30 minutes, or as long as you are comfortable.

FOOT-HEALING FOOTBATH

A footbath is one of those small pleasures in life that we rarely afford ourselves. These essential oils will have you relaxing and feeling great while imparting healing benefits throughout your feet. This recipe has therapeutic properties for quick relief such as anti-inflammatory, nervine, sedative, and analgesic agents.

Yield: 1 application

3 drops lemongrass oil
3 drops helichrysum oil
3 drops myrrh oil
1 teaspoon carrier oil
1 tablespoon milk (optional for adults,
    recommended for children)

In a container large enough to comfortably soak your feet, combine the ingredients and swirl to mix. Add warm water. Oftentimes people add 1 tablespoon milk to the water; this will cause the essential oil to blend into the water and not float on top. Soak your feet until the water is no longer a comfortable temperature. Repeat as often as needed.

PLEURISY

An infection of the lung system, usually caused by a virus, makes it very painful to breathe and takes a long period of time to recover. You must seek medical attention for any kind of chest pain. If you're diagnosed with pleurisy, medication can help. And essential oils can assist with opening the airways and controlling the pain.

Essential Oils: cypress, thyme, Roman chamomile, peppermint, oregano, eucalyptus, basil, tea tree (melaleuca), lemon, frankincense, and bergamot

DON'T MAKE ME LAUGH AIR

Run this diffuse recipe and breathe in the healing oils to help end the pain of pleurisy. This recipe contains analgesic, anti-infectious, anti-inflammatory, antiphlogistic, and mucolytic properties.

Yield: 1 application

4 drops peppermint oil
4 drops eucalyptus oil
Water

Most diffusers come with directions for using essential oils. Add the manufacturer's recommended amount of water and the oils to the diffuser and run your delightful diffuser several times a day to receive the desired effect.

LUNG RUB ME DOWN

This rub feels so good, and the essential oils permeate your body and your lungs to bring you quick and effective relief. This blend contains analgesic, antibiotic, and restorative properties.

Yield: 4 to 10 applications

4 drops bergamot oil

3 drops peppermint oil

3 drops Roman chamomile oil

2 drops basil oil

2 drops eucalyptus oil

2 ounces carrier oil

In a small container, drip the essential oils. Pour in the carrier oil and swirl to mix the oils. Rub the back and chest areas lightly with your fingertips or a soft cloth dipped into the mixture to ensure that the essential oils are distributed over the skin. You can also pour into a roll-on bottle and roll onto the desired area. Be sure not to get any into the eyes or sensitive areas. Store the remainder in a jar with a tight-fitting lid, in a cool, dark area, for up to 3 months.

FROM FOOT TO LUNG COMPRESS

Your feet absorb all of the healing benefits of these oils and disperse them throughout your body and straight to your lungs. These oils contain analgesic, antibiotic, anti-inflammatory, antispasmodic, antiviral, and stimulating properties.

YIELD: 4 TO 10 APPLICATIONS

2 drops eucalyptus oil

2 drops basil oil

2 drops cypress oil

2 ounces carrier oil

In a small container, drip the essential oils. Pour in the carrier oil and swirl to mix the oils. Apply the oil to the soles of the feet with your fingertips or a soft cloth and reapply as often as needed. Store the remainder in a jar with a tight-fitting lid, in a cool, dark area, for up to 3 months.

PMS
(Premenstrual Syndrome)

A period of time, usually the week before menses, that is marked by mood swings, bloating, fatigue, and other undesirable emotions and physical discomforts. Essential oils are derived from the plants that have been used for centuries to bring relief to women suffering from PMS, by reducing bloating and pain and helping to control mood swings.

Essential Oils: chamomile, clary sage, lavender, fennel, ylang-ylang, rosemary, helichrysum, geranium, neroli, rose, jasmine, marjoram, cypress, frankincense, tea tree (melaleuca), sandalwood, bergamot, and juniper

PMS BATH SALTS

Perfectly suited for that time of the month when you need to get away from it all, the essential oils in this recipe will help you find balance in your life. These oils contain restorative, analgesic, anti-inflammatory, antirheumatic, antispasmodic, and tonic properties.

YIELD: 5 TO 6 APPLICATIONS

7 drops tea tree (melaleuca) oil
7 drops cypress oil
7 drops rosemary oil
2 tablespoons carrier oil
3 cups salts (pink Himalayan salt, sea salt,
   Epsom salts)
1 tablespoon milk (optional for adults,
   recommended for children)

Add the oils to the salt. Stir until the mixture is well blended. Put in a jar with a lid. Let sit for 24 hours and stir again. Do not make the bathwater too hot, as the oils will dissipate. Do not add the salts when the water is running, but add ½ cup of the bath salt mixture and the milk to the water as you get into the tub. Oftentimes people add 1 tablespoon milk to the water; this will cause the essential oil to blend into the water and not float on top. Store the remainder in a jar with a tight-fitting lid, in a cool, dark area, for up to 3 months.

CALM ME DOWN BEFORE I KILL THEM BATH

The law should require this bath for every woman suffering from PMS. This perfect blend of essential oils are calming, healing, and strengthening with their antidepressant, antispasmodic, aphrodisiac, and depurative properties.

YIELD: 1 APPLICATION

5 drops chamomile oil
5 drops rose oil
5 drops clary sage oil
3 drops jasmine oil
1 tablespoon carrier oil
1 tablespoon milk (optional for adults,
   recommended for children)

While the bathwater is running, pour the ingredients into the bath. Make sure that the water is not so hot as to cause the essential oils to dissipate. Oftentimes people add 1 tablespoon milk to the water; this will cause the essential oils to blend into the water and not float on top. Soak in the water as long as you are comfortable.

TNT DIFFUSER

Have you ever felt like a stick of dynamite about to go off? Then this is the blend for you. This particular recipe is soothing and healing to the soul with its depurative, antispasmodic, antitoxic, antidepressant, anti-inflammatory, and analgesic properties.

YIELD: 1 APPLICATION

4 drops rose oil
3 drops sandalwood oil
3 drops fennel oil
2 drops juniper oil
Water

Most diffusers come with directions for using essential oils. Add the manufacturer's recommended amount of water and the oils to the diffuser and run your delightful diffuser several times a day to receive the desired effect.

INSTANT FLOODGATE RELIEF

When you're crying and unable to stop, here is the solution. These essential oils can be carried with you and used at your leisure. These oils contain antidepressant, analgesic, and anti-inflammatory properties.

YIELD: 1 APPLICATION

1 drop clary sage oil, or 1 drop geranium oil, or 1 drop rose oil

Place the drop of essential oil on a handkerchief or tissue, in the palm of your hand, or in an essential oil inhaler. Cup to your nose and inhale the aroma. Repeat several times daily or as needed.

IF YOU WANT TO LIVE, MASSAGE ME NOW!

Yep! He'd better get busy and get these essential oils on you quickly if he knows what's good for him. These PMS-reducing oils contain analgesic, antidepressant, antispasmodic, and sedative properties.

YIELD: 4 TO 10 APPLICATIONS

6 drops chamomile oil
4 drops sandalwood oil
3 drops bergamot oil
3 drops juniper oil
2 ounces carrier oil

In a small container, drip the essential oils. Pour in the carrier oil and swirl to mix the oils. Rub the back, chest, temples. and back of the neck area lightly with your fingertips or a soft cloth dipped into the mixture to ensure that the essential oils are distributed over the skin. You can also pour into a roll-on bottle and roll onto the desired area. Be sure not to get any into the eyes or sensitive areas. Store unused portion in a jar with a tight-fitting lid, in a cool, dark area, for up to 3 months.

POISON IVY/OAK/SUMAC

An allergy to various plants, which cause an extremely itchy, rashlike area on the body that can spread rapidly. There are many natural remedies for poison ivy, sumac, and oak. Essential oils can completely eradicate a poison ivy rash if the right combination is used for the right person. Ensure, using the patch test, that you do not also have an allergic reaction to these essential oils. If the rash is near any sensitive areas, it should be evaluated by a doctor.

Essential Oils: lavender, sage, chamomile, peppermint, rose, myrrh, cypress, birch, and eucalyptus

IT JUST BEGAN BANDAGE

When you spot that first itchy bump, apply this recipe and you'll get rid of that body-consuming allergy before it has a chance to spread. I use this a couple of times a year as soon as I feel that very first itch. The healing properties in this blend contain anti-inflammatory, depurative, antimicrobial, antifungal, and antibacterial properties.

YIELD: 1 APPLICATION

2 drops sage oil
2 drops lavender oil
2 drops eucalyptus oil
½ teaspoon carrier oil

Mix the ingredients well. Apply a few drops of the ingredients to a bandage or a piece of gauze with an eye dropper and secure to the site. Leave on for several hours or overnight. If any of the mixture remains, store in a container with a tight-fitting lid in the refrigerator for up to 3 days. If applying to bandage or skin, use a cotton swab or cotton ball to apply to avoid getting fingertips in oil.

CHELE'S SAGE OIL DABBER

My sister and coauthor, Chele, is highly allergic to poison ivy, poison oak, and sumac. She and her family have always had to get shots to get over it. For the past several years they have used this recipe and have not had to go to the doctor since, as this clears it up in just a couple of days. The healing properties in this blend contain anti-inflammatory, depurative, antimicrobial, antifungal, and antibacterial properties.

YIELD: 4 TO 10 APPLICATIONS

10 drops sage oil
1 ounce apple cider vinegar

Mix the ingredients and dab onto spots with an

eye dropper or cotton swab when poison ivy is first suspected. Reapply 3 to 4 times daily. Store the remainder in a jar with a tight-fitting lid, in a cool, dark area, for up to 3 months.

POISON IVY SPRAY

Use this spray on your poison ivy rash to stop the incessant itch and begin the healing process. These oils contain analgesic, antiallergenic, antibiotic, anti-infectious, and anti-inflammatory elements, to name a few.

YIELD: 50 TO 100 SPRAYS PER 4-OUNCE BOTTLE

5 drops peppermint oil
5 drops chamomile oil
4 drops lavender oil
4 drops cypress oil
4 ounces water

Combine the ingredients in a 4-ounce spray bottle, shake well, and spray the rash or itchy area. Allow to air dry. The essential oils will be absorbed into the skin by contact. Store in the spray bottle in a cool, dark area for up to 3 months.

PROSTATE PROBLEMS

Issues often arise with the prostate as a man ages. Men should have their prostate medically evaluated annually, as prostate cancer is on the rise and early detection can save lives. Essential oils can assist with recovery and soothe and relieve the prostate area.

Essential Oils: lemon, lime, clove, rosemary, helichrysum, cypress, clary sage, lavender, myrrh, oregano, and thyme

SOOTHING BATH SALTS

This calming and soothing recipe is known for its healing properties with its antispasmodic, antiseptic, euphoric, nervine, and sedative components.

YIELD: 5 TO 6 APPLICATIONS

5 drops lemon oil
5 drops rosemary oil
5 drops clary sage oil
5 drops myrrh oil
1 ounce carrier oil
3 cups salts (pink Himalayan salt, sea salt, Epsom salts)

1 tablespoon milk (optional for adults, recommended for children)

Add the oils to the salt. Stir until the mixture is well blended. Put in a jar with a lid. Let sit for 24 hours and stir again. Do not make the bathwater too hot, as the oils will dissipate. Do not add the salts when the water is running, but add ½ cup of the bath salt mixture and the milk to the water as you get into the tub. Oftentimes people add 1 tablespoon milk to the water; this will cause the essential oil to blend into the water and not float on top. Store the remainder in a jar with a tight-fitting lid, in a cool, dark area for up to 3 months.

PSORIASIS

Marked by a red and white scaly, patchy area of skin that is very itchy, psoriasis can be localized to one area or even cover most of the body. There is no cure for psoriasis, but many with psoriasis test positive for celiac disease. Allergies to other foods such as dairy, sugar, yeast, and eggs have also been known to trigger psoriasis outbreaks. Essential oils can bring soothing relief to a person suffering from psoriasis.

Essential Oils: **Roman chamomile, geranium, lavender, myrrh, lemon, frankincense, helichrysum, tea tree (melaleuca), and grapefruit**

BRIAN'S OINTMENT

These healing essential oils can soothe the dry, cracked, scaly patches that are present in eczema and psoriasis. These oils have very soothing and healing properties in them such as antibacterial, antibiotic, antifungal, anti-infectious, and anti-inflammatory agents.

YIELD: 2 TO 6 APPLICATIONS

2 drops geranium oil
2 drops tea tree (melaleuca) oil
2 drops helichrysum oil
2 drops lemon oil
1 ounce carrier oil

In a small container, drip the essential oils. Pour in the carrier oil and swirl to mix the oils. Rub the rash area lightly with your fingertips or a soft cloth dipped into the mixture to ensure that the essential oils are distributed over the skin. You can also pour into a roll-on bottle and roll onto the desired area. Be sure not to get any into the eyes or sensitive areas. Store unused portion in a jar with a tight-fitting lid, in a cool, dark area, for up to 3 months.

JENNIFER'S ITCHY RUB

When the itching from psoriasis becomes unbearable, these essential oils can bring soothing relief to get you through your day and night. The healing therapeutic properties in this blend include analgesic, antifungal, anti-inflammatory, astringent, cicatrisant, and circulatory components.

YIELD: 2 TO 6 APPLICATIONS

2 drops lavender oil
2 drops frankincense oil
2 drops grapefruit oil
2 drops myrrh oil
1 ounce carrier oil

In a small container, drip the essential oils. Pour in the carrier oil and swirl to mix the oils. Rub the desired area lightly with your fingertips or a soft cloth dipped into the mixture to ensure that the essential oils are distributed over the skin. You can also pour into a roll-on bottle and roll onto the desired area. Be sure not to get any into the eyes or sensitive areas. Store unused portion in a jar with a tight-fitting lid, in a cool, dark area, for up to 3 months.

AMANDA'S SKIN-MOISTURIZING BATH

These essential oils provide maximum relief to dry skin. The properties contained in this recipe are analgesic, antifungal, anti-inflammatory, antiseptic, astringent, and cicatrisant elements.

YIELD: 1 APPLICATION

5 drops geranium oil
5 drops tea tree (melaleuca) oil
5 drops lavender oil
1 tablespoon carrier oil
1 tablespoon milk (optional for adults, recommended for children)

While the bathwater is running, pour the essential oils and carrier oil into the bath. Make sure that the water is not so hot as to cause the essential oils to dissipate. Oftentimes people add 1 tablespoon milk to the water; this will cause the essential oils to blend into the water and not float on top. Soak in the water as long as you are comfortable.

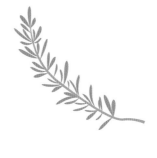

PULMONARY CONDITIONS

The lungs can be host to many diseases, viruses, and bacteria. Medical attention should be sought immediately when it is suspected that the lungs have been compromised. Essential oils can bring relief and easier breathing to a person with chronic or minor lung disease or illness, along with care from their physician. Ensure through your physician that these essential oils will not interfere with your medications.

Essential Oils: cardamom, eucalyptus, frankincense, sandalwood, wild orange, ravensara, peppermint, clove, oregano, and lemon

TEENA'S FRESH AIR

This light diffuse recipe is great for people who cannot stand strong smells and need a light diffuser with healing properties for the lungs. The healing elements in this blend include analgesic, antibacterial, antifungal, anti-inflammatory, antispasmodic, decongestant, and expectorant properties.

YIELD: 1 APPLICATION

2 drops cardamom oil

2 drops peppermint oil
2 drops ravensara oil
1 drop eucalyptus oil
Water

Most diffusers come with directions for using essential oils. Add the manufacturer's recommended amount of water and the oils to the diffuser and run your delightful diffuser several times a day to receive the desired effect.

ASHLEY'S BREATHE BETTER INHALER

Lungs open and feel great after inhaling a bit of the aroma from one of these essential oils with their decongestant and expectorant properties.

YIELD: 1 APPLICATION

1 drop eucalyptus oil, or 1 drop frankincense oil, or 1 drop lemon oil, or 1 drop peppermint oil

Place the drop of essential oil on a handkerchief or tissue, in the palm of your hand, or in an essential oil inhaler. Cup to your nose and inhale the aroma. Repeat several times daily or as needed.

RASH

Rashes take as many different forms as there are reasons to have a rash. Often it is just a reaction to a chemical or an outside agent. Some rashes last a few minutes, others seem to last a lifetime. A physician can help you determine the cause of your rash and provide treatment in many cases. Essential oils can help to soothe and stop the itch that accompanies many rashes.

Essential Oils: helichrysum, lavender, geranium, clary sage, basil, sandalwood, Roman chamomile, thyme, rose, peppermint, myrrh, tea tree (melaleuca), oregano, and eucalyptus

JESSE'S SPOT-ON RASH TREATMENT

This rub uses the essential oils that work best for redness, drying skin, and itching. The active ingredients in this rash are antiseptic, astringent, bactericidal, and moisturizing agents.

YIELD: 2 TO 6 APPLICATIONS

1 drop tea tree (melaleuca) oil
1 drop clary sage oil
1 drop basil oil
1 drop geranium oil
1 ounce carrier oil

In a small container, drip the essential oils. Pour in the carrier oil and swirl to mix the oils. Rub the rash area lightly with your fingertips or a soft cloth dipped into the mixture to ensure that the essential oils are distributed over the skin. You can also pour into a roll-on bottle and roll onto the desired area. Be sure not to get any into the eyes or sensitive areas. Store unused portion in a jar with a tight-fitting lid, in a cool, dark area, for up to 3 months.

ANGELA'S ITCH SPRITZ

Spraying this recipe on an itchy rash will end the itching in no time with its anesthetic, anti-inflammatory, and astringent properties.

YIELD: 25 TO 50 SPRAYS PER 2-OUNCE BOTTLE

3 drops lavender oil
3 drops helichrysum oil
3 drops peppermint oil
3 drops Roman chamomile oil
2 ounces water

Combine the oils and water in a 4-ounce spray bottle. Lightly spritz onto the itchy area. Allow to air dry. The essential oils will be absorbed by the skin on contact. Store in the spray bottle in a cool, dark area for up to 3 months.

VANCE'S SKIN-SOOTHING BATH

The essential oils used in this bath will soothe your itchy skin and moisturize your body as well as promote healing. The healing agents at work here include antifungal, antimicrobial, anti-inflammatory, and astringent properties, among others.

YIELD: 1 APPLICATION

3 drops tea tree (melaleuca) oil
3 drops lavender oil
3 drops clary sage oil
3 drops geranium oil
3 drops sandalwood oil
1 tablespoon carrier oil
1 tablespoon milk (optional for adults, recommended for children)

While the bathwater is running, pour the ingredients into the bath. Make sure that the water is not so hot as to cause the essential oils to dissipate. Oftentimes people add 1 tablespoon milk to the water; this will cause the essential oils to blend into the water and not float on top. Soak in the water as long as you are comfortable.

RESPIRATORY INFECTION

A respiratory infection is often a medical emergency and must be treated by a physician. During the recovery process, essential oils can be used to speed the healing process, relax the patient, and make breathing less labored. Ensure, through your physician, that your medications and the oils can be used together.

Essential Oils: peppermint, eucalyptus, tea tree (melaleuca), clove, lemon, wild orange, benzoin, lavender, marjoram, cinnamon, frankincense, thyme, sandalwood, and oregano

ENERGETIC INHALE

When lack of oxygen from respiratory ailments have you feeling tired and listless, try inhaling a whiff of one of these essential oils for a quick pick-me-up! These oils contain, in part, analgesic, tonic, anti-inflammatory, and expectorant properties.

YIELD: 1 APPLICATION

1 drop peppermint oil, or 1 drop tea tree (melaleuca) oil

Place the drop of essential oil on a handkerchief or tissue, in the palm of your hand, or in an essential oil inhaler. Cup to your nose and inhale the aroma. Repeat several times daily or as needed.

DEEP BREAK-UP RUB

These essential oils have congestion-fighting properties. Use this rub on your back and chest to break up that mucus and get you breathing well again with their anti-inflammatory, decongestant, expectorant, and analgesic properties.

YIELD: 2 TO 6 APPLICATIONS

2 drops peppermint oil
2 drops lavender oil
2 drops eucalyptus oil
2 drops tea tree (melaleuca) oil
1 ounce carrier oil

In a small container, drip the essential oils. Pour in the carrier oil and swirl to mix the oils. Rub the desired area lightly with your fingertips or a soft cloth dipped into the mixture to ensure that the essential oils are distributed over the skin. You can also pour into a roll-on bottle and roll onto the desired area. Be sure not to get any into the eyes or sensitive areas. Store unused portion in a jar with a tight-fitting lid, in a cool, dark area, for up to 3 months.

HOOVER'S HELPFUL MASSAGE

This massage will relax the patient and also get them breathing better with its therapeutic and healing essential oils. A few of the properties in these oils are expectorant, analgesic, antispasmodic, and antiphlogistic.

YIELD: 4 TO 10 APPLICATIONS

4 drops frankincense oil
3 drops peppermint oil
2 drops marjoram oil
2 drops lemon oil
2 ounces carrier oil

In a small container, drip the essential oils. Pour in the carrier oil and swirl to mix the oils. Rub the lung, chest, and back areas lightly with your fingertips or a soft cloth dipped into the mixture to ensure that the essential oils are distributed over the skin. You can also pour into a roll-on bottle and roll onto the desired area. Be sure not to get any into the eyes or sensitive areas. Store the remainder in a jar with a tight-fitting lid, in a cool, dark area, for up to 3 months.

RESTLESS LEG SYNDROME

Many studies point to a lack of vitamins, specifically iron, as the primary cause of RLS, which some people can experience several times a night. I suffered from RLS for thirty years until a doctor told me to buy some cheap iron pills for my anemia. I did, and I noticed that for two nights in a row I didn't have RLS. Now I keep a bottle of iron pills by my bed, and as soon as my leg moves I take one. Miraculous! If I have too much bad food, the iron pills won't help, so I use these essential oils to help me get to sleep and stay asleep.

Essential Oils: lavender, frankincense, marjoram, and Roman chamomile

STOP MOVING LEG MASSAGE

Keep this recipe handy by your bed and apply liberally when those jerky leg movements repeatedly wake you up. These essential oils are full of healing properties that can help you regain sleep. Components in this blend include sedative, nervine, and analgesic agents.

YIELD: 4 TO 10 APPLICATIONS

6 drops frankincense oil
4 drops Roman chamomile oil
3 drops lavender oil
3 drops marjoram oil
2 ounces carrier oil

In a small container, drip the essential oils. Pour in the carrier oil and swirl to mix the oils. Rub the leg and ankle areas lightly with your fingertips or a soft cloth dipped into the mixture to ensure that the essential oils are distributed over the skin. You can also pour into a roll-on bottle and roll onto the desired area. Be sure not to get any into the eyes or sensitive areas. Store the remainder in a jar with a tight-fitting lid, in a cool, dark area, for up to 3 months.

RHEUMATOID ARTHRITIS

A crippling and disabling disease of the joints, tendons, muscles, and connective tissues. This can be a life-altering disease, as it can lead to mobility issues, but many believe that with medications, exercise, and diet, it can be kept under control. Essential oils can bring relief to the joints and areas affected by rheumatoid arthritis when applied through massages, baths, and rubs.

Essential Oils: ginger, birch, lavender, lemon, eucalyptus, lime, German chamomile, marjoram, helichrysum, black pepper, frankincense, myrrh, oregano, peppermint, vetiver, basil, geranium, sandalwood, ylang-ylang, lemongrass, niaouli, juniper, fennel, cypress, clove, cinnamon, cedarwood, benzoin, rosemary, and camphor

RHEUMATOID BATH SALTS

In this bath, not only will the salts provide relief to your aching bones, but the essential oils have healing properties that will hasten you toward healthy living. The healing properties include analgesic, anti-inflammatory, antirheumatic, antispasmodic, and relaxant components.

Yield: 5 to 6 applications

7 drops rosemary oil
7 drops niaouli oil
7 drops German chamomile oil
5 drops lavender oil
1 ounce carrier oil
3 cups salts (pink Himalayan salt, sea salt, Epsom salts)
1 tablespoon milk (optional for adults, recommended for children)

Add the oils to the salt. Stir until the mixture is well blended. Put in a jar with a lid. Let sit for 24 hours and stir again. Do not make the bathwater too hot, as the oils will dissipate. Do not add the salts when the water is running, but add ½ cup of the bath salt mixture and the milk to the water as you get into the tub. Oftentimes people add 1 tablespoon milk to the water; this will cause the essential oil to blend into the water and not float on top. Store the remainder in a jar with a tight-fitting lid, in a cool, dark area, for up to 3 months.

MICHELE'S RHEUMATOID RUB

This particular rub is so helpful to my sister who suffers from rheumatoid arthritis. She likes to rub this on in the morning after a bad night of deep aches and pains. This recipe contains restorative, anti-inflammatory, antirheumatic, nervine, analgesic, sedative, and revitalizing properties.

Yield: 2 to 6 applications

3 drops lavender oil
2 drops basil oil
2 drops cedarwood oil
2 drops myrrh oil
2 drops lemongrass oil
1 ounce carrier oil

In a small container, drip the essential oils. Pour in the carrier oil and swirl to mix the oils. Rub the desired area lightly with your fingertips or a soft cloth dipped into the mixture to ensure that the essential oils are distributed over the skin. You can also pour into a roll-on bottle and roll onto the desired area. Be sure not to get any into the eyes or sensitive areas. Store unused portion in a jar with a tight-fitting lid, in a cool, dark area, for up to 3 months.

DIANE'S DELICIOUS BATH

This bath will help your loved one enjoy a relaxing, healing, soothing time while the essential oils bring them wonderful aromas and good health. The healing components in this bath include nervine, antirheumatic, sedative, antispasmodic, analgesic, anti-inflammatory, and tranquilizing properties.

YIELD: 1 APPLICATION

3 drops frankincense oil
3 drops ginger oil
3 drops ylang-ylang oil
3 drops vetiver oil
3 drops lavender oil
1 tablespoon carrier oil
1 tablespoon milk (optional for adults,
*   recommended for children)*

While the bathwater is running, pour the ingredients into the bath. Make sure that the water is not so hot as to cause the essential oils to dissipate. Oftentimes people add 1 tablespoon milk to the water; this will cause the essential oils to blend into the water and not float on top. Soak in the water as long as you are comfortable.

Note: Alternatively, you can use 2 drops of each of the above oils in a bucket of water and soak your hands and feet to gain relief.

RINGWORM

Actually, this is not a worm; it's a contagious fungus. Ringworm can attack any area of the body and is most prevalent among school-age children. For centuries the plants from which we extract these essential oils have helped to end the itch associated with ringworm.

Essential Oils: geranium, oregano, peppermint, myrrh, thyme, tea tree (melaleuca), lavender, manuka, lemon, eucalyptus, and cypress

RINGWORM BANDAGE

This is best used when you first notice the ringworm. These essential oils will stop the fungus in its tracks with the antibacterial, antifungal, fungicidal, and anti-inflammatory properties.

YIELD: 1 APPLICATION

2 drops oregano oil
2 drops tea tree (melaleuca) oil
2 drops lavender oil
½ teaspoon carrier oil

Mix the ingredients well. Apply a few drops of the ingredients to a bandage or a piece of gauze with your fingertips or a cotton swab and secure to the site. Leave on for several hours or overnight. If any of the mixture remains, store in a container with a tight-fitting lid in the refrigerator for up to 3 days. If applying to a bandage or skin, use a cotton swab or cotton ball to apply to avoid getting fingertips in the oil.

DAB IT ROUND

When the ringworm starts spreading, apply this rub over the entire area to prevent further spreading and to heal the places that are already affected. This blend contains antifungal, anti-inflammatory, antitoxic, and fungicidal therapeutic properties.

YIELD: 2 TO 6 APPLICATIONS

3 drops geranium oil
2 drops oregano oil

2 drops thyme oil
1 ounce carrier oil

In a small container, drip the essential oils. Pour in the carrier oil and swirl to mix the oils. Rub the desired area lightly with your fingertips or a soft cloth dipped into the mixture to ensure that the essential oils are distributed over the skin. You can also pour into a roll-on bottle and roll onto the desired area. Be sure not to get any into the eyes or sensitive areas. Store unused portion in a jar with a tight-fitting lid, in a cool, dark area, for up to 3 months.

KILL THE RINGWORM NOW

These essential oils are reputed to kill ringworm after applying the mixture repeatedly for a few days. The healing elements in this blend include antifungal, analgesic, fungicidal, anti-inflammatory, and cicatrisant properties.

YIELD: 2 TO 6 APPLICATIONS

2 drops tea tree (melaleuca) oil
2 drops geranium oil
2 drops oregano oil
1 ounce carrier oil

In a small container, drip the essential oils. Pour in the carrier oil and swirl to mix the oils. Rub the desired area lightly with your fingertips or a soft cloth dipped into the mixture to ensure that the essential oils are distributed over the skin. You can also pour into a roll-on bottle and roll onto the desired area. Be sure not to get any into the eyes or sensitive areas. Store unused portion in a jar with a tight-fitting lid, in a cool, dark area, for up to 3 months.

ROSACEA

Rosacea causes redness of the skin across the face, primarily in women. Essential oils can be used to help treat rosacea, smooth your complexion, and prevent further damage to the skin. Certain skin-care lines also have medications in them to diminish the appearance of rosacea.

Essential Oils: frankincense, helichrysum, rosemary, sandalwood, and lavender

MICHALA'S FACE SPRAY

These essential oils will heal the rough redness of rosacea and smooth out your skin tone and color. The healing elements in this blend include anti-inflammatory, antiseptic, astringent, cicatrisant, and emollient agents. Do not spray in the eyes or mouth.

YIELD: 25 TO 50 SPRAYS PER 2-OUNCE BOTTLE

3 drops sandalwood oil

3 drops frankincense oil

3 drops lavender oil

2 drops helichrysum oil

2 ounces water

Combine the ingredients in a 2-ounce spray bottle and lightly spray the affected area. Allow to air dry. The essential oils will be absorbed into the skin by contact. You can also dab the mixture onto the affected area with your fingertips or a cotton ball. Store in the spray bottle in a cool, dark area for up to 3 months.

SCABIES

An infection of the skin caused by tiny mites, scabies present as red, silvery lines that itch where the mites burrow under the skin. Essential oils are extremely effective in treating scabies, and are derived from plants and herbs that have been used for centuries in fighting these little pests.

Essential Oils: lavender, tea tree (melaleuca), peppermint, bergamot, oregano, cinnamon, clove, thyme, rosemary, pine, and lemongrass

SCABIES BANDAGE

This recipe works best when you first notice the scabies. The elements to heal and protect you are antibacterial, antifungal, anti-infectious, antimicrobial, antiparasitic, balsamic, and insecticidal properties.

YIELD: 1 APPLICATION

2 drops tea tree (melaleuca) oil
2 drops lavender oil
½ teaspoon carrier oil

Mix the ingredients well. Apply a few drops to a bandage or a piece of gauze with an eye dropper or a cotton swab and secure to the site. Leave on for several hours or overnight. If any of the mixture remains, store in a container with a tight-fitting lid in the refrigerator for up to 3 days. If applying to a bandage or skin, use a cotton swab or cotton ball to apply to avoid getting fingertips in the oil.

SCABIES SPRAY

Use this spray on bedding, carpets, blankets, pillows, and even clothing. The healing elements include antibacterial, antifungal, anti-infectious, antimicrobial, antiparasitic, balsamic, and insecticidal properties.

YIELD: 50 TO 100 SPRAYS PER 4-OUNCE BOTTLE

5 drops tea tree (melaleuca) oil
3 drops thyme oil
3 drops peppermint oil
4 ounces water

Combine the ingredients in a 4-ounce spray bottle and lightly spray the affected area. Allow to air dry. The essential oils will be absorbed into the skin by contact. Store in the spray bottle in a cool, dark area for up to 3 months.

ITCH-RELIEF BATH

The essential oils in this bath recipe will bring instant relief to the incessant itching. The medicinal ingredients in this blend include antibacterial, antifungal, anti-infectious, antimicrobial, antiparasitic, balsamic, and insecticidal properties.

YIELD: 1 APPLICATION

4 drops lavender oil
4 drops tea tree (melaleuca) oil
4 drops bergamot oil
2 drops lemongrass oil
1 tablespoon carrier oil
1 tablespoon milk (optional for adults,
*   recommended for children)*

While the bathwater is running, pour the ingredients into the bath. Make sure that the water is not so hot as to cause the essential oils to dissi-

pate. Oftentimes people add 1 tablespoon milk to the water; this will cause the essential oils to blend into the water and not float on top. Soak in the water as long as you are comfortable.

SCARS

When the skin is damaged, the body repairs itself. Scars are the fibrous tissues that result from that repair. Essential oils have long been used to reduce the appearance of scars and redness and sometimes even to prevent a scar from forming.

Essential Oils: frankincense, lavender, yarrow, patchouli, helichrysum, eucalyptus, geranium, palmarosa, neroli, mandarin, white fir, sandalwood, rose, and myrrh

SCAR BANDAGE

This recipe will prevent scarring if applied to a healed wound with its anti-inflammatory, antiseptic, astringent, cicatrisant, and cytophylactic properties.

Yield: 1 application

2 drops frankincense oil

1 drop helichrysum oil
1 drop lavender oil
½ teaspoon carrier oil

Mix the ingredients well. Apply a few drops of the ingredients to a bandage or a piece of gauze with an eye dropper or a cotton swab and secure to the site. Leave on for several hours or overnight. Reapply daily or as needed. If any of the mixture remains, store in a container with a tight-fitting lid in the refrigerator for up to 3 days. If applying to a bandage or skin, use a cotton swab or cotton ball to apply to avoid getting fingertips in the oil.

NO-SCAR RUB

These essential oils can even out the skin tone of some scars and make them less pronounced. The healing agents in this blend include anti-inflammatory, antiseptic, astringent, cicatrisant, and cytophylactic properties.

Yield: 2 to 6 applications

2 drops helichrysum oil
2 drops frankincense oil
1 drop geranium oil
1 ounce carrier oil

In a small container, drip the essential oils. Pour in the carrier oil and swirl to mix the oils. Rub the scar and surrounding area lightly with your fingertips or a soft cloth dipped into the mixture to ensure that the essential oils are distributed over the skin. You can also pour into a roll-on bottle and roll onto the desired area. Be sure not to get any into the eyes or sensitive areas. Store unused portion in a jar with a tight-fitting lid, in a cool, dark area, for up to 3 months.

PALMAROSA SCAR RUB

These essential oils have been used for years to reduce the redness and bumpiness of scars. The healing elements in this blend contain antiseptic, bactericidal, anti-inflammatory, cytophylactic, hydrating, and astringent properties, among others.

Yield: 2 to 6 applications

3 drops palmarosa oil
3 drops patchouli oil
2 drops white fir oil
2 drops myrtle oil
1 ounce carrier oil

In a small container, drip the essential oils. Pour in the carrier oil and swirl to mix the oils. Rub the scar area lightly with your fingertips or a soft cloth dipped into the mixture to ensure that the essential oils are distributed over the skin. You can also pour into a roll-on bottle and roll onto the desired area. Be sure not to get any into the eyes or sensitive areas. Store unused portion in

a jar with a tight-fitting lid, in a cool, dark area, for up to 3 months.

SINUSITIS

A very common condition that affects millions of people annually, sinusitis can be caused by allergies, viruses, or other factors. Essential oils can be used to relieve pain, fight infections, decrease mucus, and help the healing process. If symptoms are severe or continue for more than a few days, consult a doctor.

Essential Oils: peppermint, eucalyptus, pine, basil, thyme, tea tree (melaleuca), clove, hyssop, spearmint, niaouli, myrrh, rosemary, geranium, ginger, lavender, white fir, and linden blossom

SINUS-DRAINING STEAM

The essential oils in this steam will drain your sinuses and bring you relief quickly with their anesthetic, analgesic, anti-infectious, anti-inflammatory, and decongestant properties. Do not use this around children, as they may tip the pan of water and burn themselves.

Yield: 1 application

4 drops peppermint oil
4 drops eucalyptus oil
2 drops rosemary oil
1 bowl hot water

Combine the oils in the bowl of hot water. Be careful not to spill water on yourself. Place a towel over your head and drape it over the bowl. Breathe deeply of the steam that rises until the water cools. Discard the mixture after use.

CLEAR SINUS AIR

This diffuse recipe will help you to breathe easier and go about your busy day. The healing elements of this recipe are analgesic, antibacterial, antifungal, anti-inflammatory, antimicrobial, and expectorant properties.

YIELD: 1 APPLICATION

3 drops eucalyptus oil
3 drops frankincense oil
2 drops lavender oil
Water

Most diffusers come with directions for using essential oils. Add the manufacturer's recommended amount of water and the oils to the diffuser and run your delightful diffuser several times a day to receive the desired effect.

HEAVEN'S MASSAGE

When feeling clogged up and unable to even focus on anything, this massage will bring it all back into perspective for you by relieving the pain and clearing the inflammation. A few of the healing agents in this recipe include analgesic, antispasmodic, anti-inflammatory, sudorific, and bactericidal properties.

YIELD: 4 TO 10 APPLICATIONS

3 drops peppermint oil
3 drops lemon oil
3 drops ginger oil
2 drops linden blossom oil
2 drops hyssop oil
2 ounces carrier oil

In a small container, drip the essential oils. Pour in the carrier oil and swirl to mix the oils. Rub the outer sinus area and cheek area lightly with your fingertips or a soft cloth dipped into the mixture to ensure that the essential oils are distributed over the skin. You can also pour into a roll-on bottle and roll onto the desired area. Be sure not to get any into the eyes or sensitive areas. This can be repeated as needed. Store the remainder in a jar with a tight-fitting lid, in a cool, dark area, for up to 3 months.

SKIN TAGS

These are benign tumors that often grow in the folds of the skin. They are usually harmless—consult a dermatologist to be sure—but they can be annoying if they're in a place where you shave, wear clothing, or have a skin rash. Essential oils can be used to eradicate some skin tags, when used regularly.

Essential Oils: oregano, helichrysum, Roman chamomile, ylang-ylang, cypress, frankincense, patchouli, sandalwood, peppermint, myrrh, lemon, geranium, and lavender

TAG BANDAGE

I used oregano oil on the skin tag on my own neck. It just got smaller and smaller until one day I noticed it was gone! The first time I used it, I just put the oregano oil on neat: big mistake! It really burned my neck, so I learned quickly to always mix it with carrier oil. The healing elements in this recipe include analgesic, anti-inflammatory, antitoxic, antiviral, and tonic properties.

Yield: 1 application

3 drops oregano oil
½ teaspoon carrier oil

Mix the ingredients well. Apply a few drops of the mixture to a bandage or a piece of gauze with a cotton swab and secure to the site. Leave on for several hours or overnight. If any of the mixture remains, store in a container with a tight-fitting lid in the refrigerator for up to 3 days. If applying to a bandage or skin, use a cotton swab or cotton ball to apply to avoid getting fingertips in the oil.

GET THE %&$ OFF ME!

A few of the agents in this skin tag terminator include anti-inflammatory, antiseptic, antiviral, cicatrisant, and tonic properties.

Yield: 2 to 6 applications

4 drops helichrysum oil
3 drops oregano oil
1 ounce carrier oil

In a small container, drip the essential oils. Pour in the carrier oil and swirl to mix the oils. Rub the skin tag lightly with your fingertips or a soft cloth dipped into the mixture to ensure that the essential oils are distributed over the skin. You can also pour into a roll-on bottle and roll onto the desired area. Be sure not to get any into the eyes or sensitive areas. Store unused portion in a jar with a tight-fitting lid, in a cool, dark area, for up to 3 months.

SHRINK IT AWAY

This recipe contains skin tag–shrinking essential oils that will work wonders on deleting that foreign invader. The fighting elements include anti-infectious, anti-inflammatory, antiseptic, astringent, and restorative properties.

YIELD: 2 TO 6 APPLICATIONS

3 drops frankincense oil
2 drops cypress oil
1 ounce carrier oil

In a small container, drip the essential oils. Pour in the carrier oil and swirl to mix the oils. Rub the desired area lightly with your fingertips or a soft cloth dipped into the mixture to ensure that the essential oils are distributed over the skin. You can also pour into a roll-on bottle and roll onto the desired area. Be sure not to get any into the eyes or sensitive areas. Store unused portion in a jar with a tight-fitting lid, in a cool, dark area, for up to 3 months.

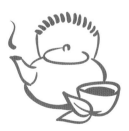

SLEEP APNEA

People with sleep apnea usually don't know it unless someone tells them. While asleep, the person's breathing stops, then he or she briefly wakes to take a breath, then falls back to sleep. This can leave someone fatigued for years without realizing why. If a medical professional has diagnosed you with sleep apnea, essential oils can help reduce your symptoms by opening the airways and allowing for easier breathing.

Essential Oils: lemon, lime, grapefruit, orange, wild orange, sandalwood, frankincense, thyme, ylang-ylang, and lavender

APNEA FOOT RUB

These essential oils have long been known to help people end the sleep-interrupting cycle. A few of the healing and sleep-inducing properties in this recipe are antispasmodic, expectorant, tonic, sedative, detoxifying, and tranquilizing.

YIELD: 2 TO 6 APPLICATIONS

2 drops thyme oil
2 drops frankincense oil
2 drops vetiver oil
2 drops lemon oil
1 ounce carrier oil

Mix the ingredients together. Apply oil to the soles of the feet with your fingertips or a cotton ball nightly or as often as needed. Store unused portion in a jar with a tight-fitting lid, in a cool, dark area, for up to 3 months.

SMELL, LOSS OF
(Anosmia)

There are many possible reasons for losing one's sense of smell, the most common being a head injury, which should always be evaluated by a medical professional. Colds, ear and sinus infections, and upper respiratory ailments are some of the simplest reasons you could lose your sense of smell. Essential oils can help bring back a sense of smell in at least one nostril.

Essential Oils: basil, tea tree (melaleuca), peppermint, rosemary, lime, orange, and lemon

SMELL THAT SMELL

Peppermint oil, when used over time, has been known to restore one's sense of smell, even if the person hasn't smelled anything very well for a long time. The invigorating, restorative, and tonic properties in peppermint oils are said to be so strong that even a nonsmeller can smell them. Give it a try, it can't hurt!

YIELD: 1 APPLICATION

1 drop peppermint oil

Place the drop of essential oil on a handkerchief or tissue, in the palm of your hand, or in an essential oil inhaler. Cup to your nose and inhale the aroma. Repeat several times daily or as needed.

NOSTRIL RUB

Essential oils have been used for a long time to help people redevelop their sense of smell once it has been lost. This recipe has worked wonders with its revitalizing, restorative, and tonic agents.

YIELD: 1 APPLICATION

1 drop rosemary oil
1 drop basil oil
1 drop tea tree (melaleuca) oil
1 drop lemon oil
1 teaspoon carrier oil

In a small container, drip the essential oils. Pour in the carrier oil and swirl to mix the oils. Rub the desired area lightly with your fingertips or a soft cloth dipped into the mixture to ensure that the essential oils are distributed over the skin. You can also pour into a roll-on bottle and roll onto the desired area. Be sure not to get any into the eyes or sensitive areas. If any of the mixture remains, store in a container with a tight-fitting lid in the refrigerator for up to 3 days.

SMOKING, QUITTING

One of the best things you can do for your body is to stop smoking, dipping, or using tobacco in any form. When quitting, a person can become agitated, angry, depressed, melancholy, and nearly every emotion under the sun. Essential oils can assist by conveying a sense of peace and calm during the withdrawal process. Some essential oils are reputed to even help curb the cravings associated with tobacco withdrawal. I used these essential oils while quitting smoking after forty years of the habit, and have had great success for five years.

Essential Oils: black pepper, clove, lemon, lime, orange, cilantro, cinnamon, grapefruit, vetiver, lavender, and ylang-ylang

WITHDRAWAL POWDER

Nighttime is a hard time when you are trying to quit smoking. The essential oils in this recipe are great for lulling yourself into a peaceful sleep. The sleep-promoting properties included in this blend are, in part, antidepressant, restorative, sedative, and detoxifying.

YIELD: 10 TO 20 APPLICATIONS

3 drops lavender oil
3 drops vetiver oil
3 drops ylang-ylang oil
¼ cup cornstarch

Combine the ingredients very well with a whisk. Pour into a mason jar with holes poked into the lid. Shake the powder inside a pillowcase or under the sheets, and wake up in the morning with renewed energy after a cool, peaceful night's sleep. When storing your jar, you can place a piece of plastic wrap under the lid so that the powder won't spill out of the jar. Store in a jar with a tight-fitting lid, in a cool, dark, dry area, for up to 3 months.

STOP SMOKING BATH SALTS

Infuse your skin with these essential oils reputed to end nicotine cravings. The healing elements in this blend include antidepressant, aphrodisiac, euphoric, hypotensive, nervine, and sedative properties.

YIELD: 5 TO 6 APPLICATIONS

7 drops ylang-ylang oil
7 drops cilantro oil
7 drops citrus oil (such as lemon, lime or orange oil)
2 tablespoon carrier oil
3 cups salts (pink Himalayan salt, sea salt, Epsom salts)
1 tablespoon milk (optional for adults, recommended for children)

Add the oils to the salt. Stir until the mixture is well blended. Put in a jar with a lid. Let sit for 24 hours and stir again. Do not make the bathwater too hot, as the oils will dissipate. Do not add the salts when the water is running, but add ½ cup of the bath salt mixture and the milk to the water as you get into the tub. Oftentimes people add 1 tablespoon milk to the water; this will cause the essential oil to blend into the water and not float on top. Store the remainder in a jar with a tight-fitting lid, in a cool, dark area, for up to 3 months.

INHALE GOOD OVER EVIL

Inhaling the aroma of these essential oils can stop nicotine cravings in their tracks. The heal-ing elements in these oils include tonic, anti-oxidant, anti-inflammatory, stimulating, and detoxifying elements.

YIELD: 1 APPLICATION

1 drop black pepper oil, or 1 drop clove oil, or 1 drop citrus oil (such as lemon, lime, or orange oil), or 1 drop cinnamon oil

Place the drop of essential oil on a handkerchief or tissue, in the palm of your hand, or in an essential oil inhaler. Cup to your nose and inhale the aroma. Repeat several times daily or as needed.

SNORING

Snoring doesn't bother the person who is doing it as much as the person sleeping next to them! Essential oils have been known to assist greatly in reducing or eliminating snoring in many people. Try several different recipes until you find the one that works best for you.

Essential Oils: wild orange, lavender, thyme, marjoram, eucalyptus, and cypress

SILENCE POWDER

Your partner won't know that you are using this powder for any reason other than the great aroma. But actually, the healing properties of these oils open the passageways and allow for easier breathing and a better night's sleep with their antispasmodic and anti-inflammatory components.

YIELD: 10 TO 20 APPLICATIONS

3 drops cypress oil
3 drops lavender oil
3 drops eucalyptus oil
¼ cup cornstarch

Combine the ingredients very well with a whisk. Pour into a mason jar with holes poked into the lid. Shake the powder inside a pillowcase or under the sheets, and wake up in the morning with renewed energy after a cool, peaceful, quiet night's sleep. When storing your jar, you can place a piece of plastic wrap under the lid so that the powder won't spill out of the jar. Store in a jar with a tight-fitting lid, in a cool, dark, dry area, for up to 3 months.

FOOT RUB

The essential oils in this foot rub recipe have long been used to stop snoring and for breathing. The soles of the feet have been proven to transport essential oil properties to every cell in the body within just a few minutes. The healing properties in this blend include sedative, restorative, antispasmodic, hypertensive, and expectorant agents.

YIELD: 1 APPLICATION

2 drops thyme oil
2 drops lavender oil
1 teaspoon carrier oil

Mix the ingredients together in a small container. Apply the oil to the soles of the feet with your fingertips and reapply as often as needed.

VANCE'S AIR

This is my personal favorite essential oils diffuser to run at night to ease my husband's snoring. It works! The healing properties in this little recipe include antidepressant, antispasmodic, aphrodisiac, tonic, and sedative elements.

YIELD: 1 APPLICATION

2 drops eucalyptus oil
2 drops marjoram oil
1 drop wild orange oil
Water

Most diffusers come with directions for using essential oils. Add the manufacturer's recommended amount of water and the oils to the diffuser and run your delightful diffuser several times a day to receive the desired effect.

SORE THROAT

There are so many causes for a sore throat: illness, allergies, strep, contamination, chemicals, and the list goes on. If a sore throat is severe or lasts more than a couple of days, you must seek medical attention. For a mild sore throat, essential oils can relieve the pain and difficulty of breathing with the mouth open. Gargles are a great way to reduce the redness and pain.

Essential Oils: thieves', oregano, sandalwood, hyssop, lemon, lavender, marjoram, tea tree (melaleuca), bergamot, and sage

QUIET TIME RUB

This recipe uses essential oils that fight inflammation of the throat and ease pain. Some of the healing properties in this blend include analgesic, antiseptic, antispasmodic, antiviral, and bactericidal elements.

YIELD: 1 TO 2 APPLICATIONS

3 drops thieves' oil
2 drops marjoram oil
2 drops sage oil
1 tablespoon carrier oil

Mix the ingredients together in a small container. Apply the oil to the soles of the feet with your fingertips and rub as often as needed. Store the remainder in a jar with a tight-fitting lid, in a cool, dark area, for up to 1 month.

THROAT WRAP

As a small child, anytime someone in the family had a sore throat or any type of upper respiratory illness, the women in the family would bring out the "Sally rag." This, to me, was a very comforting, special piece of magic. I would fall asleep quickly after inhaling the strange scents in the Sally rag, and sleep well all night. Chances are that the medicines they used in their concoctions were from the plants and herbs that these essential oils were derived from. A few of the healing properties in these oils contain antibacterial, antibiotic, antifungal, anti-infectious, anti-inflammatory, and decongestant ingredients.

YIELD: 1 APPLICATION

2 drops lavender oil
2 drops bergamot oil

1 drop tea tree (melaleuca) oil
1 drop eucalyptus oil
1 cloth

Using an eye dropper, drip the oils onto the cloth and fold the cloth lengthwise. Apply the cloth to the neck by tucking it inside the front or back of the pajama top.

I CAN SWALLOW GARGLE

This is the go-to gargle in our home when a sore throat first makes its appearance. Just gargle and spit. The healing effects of the oils are felt immediately with their astringent, detoxifying, tonic, analgesic, antiseptic, and antiviral properties.

YIELD: 1 TO 2 APPLICATIONS

2 drops marjoram oil
2 drops lemon oil
½ cup warm water
½ teaspoon salt

Ensure that your essential oil is safe for consumption and internal use and is clinical/therapeutic grade. Mix the ingredients in a small cup. Swish in the mouth or gargle, then spit it out. Repeat 3 or 4 times daily until your throat feels better. Store unused portion in a jar with a tight-fitting lid, in a cool, dark area or the refrigerator, for up to 1 day.

SPLINTER

For those tiny splinters that you just can't get with the tweezers, essential oils can be used to draw the splinter out. Soak a bandage, gauze pad, or compress with the oils and adhere it to the splinter for several hours.

Essential Oils: frankincense, helichrysum, lemon, geranium, myrrh, tea tree (melaleuca), and lavender

SPLINTER SUCKER

These essential oils apparently have the ability to draw out splinters. Use this recipe to get that splinter that you can't quite grasp with tweezers. Its properties can also heal that wound up quickly, including analgesic, anti-inflammatory, antiseptic, astringent, cicatrisant, cytophylactic, and antiviral agents.

YIELD: 1 APPLICATION

1 drop helichrysum oil
1 drop frankincense oil
5 drops carrier oil

Mix the ingredients with an eye dropper, apply to a bandage, and tape securely to the site. Leave on for several hours or overnight. Carefully remove the bandage and withdraw the splinter.

OIL DRAW

Blending these oils together brings out their drawing power. They also have amazing healing powers such as analgesic, antibacterial, cicatrisan, and antiseptic properties, which will take care of that wound after the splinter is out.

YIELD: 1 APPLICATION

1 drop tea tree (melaleuca) oil
1 drop lavender oil

Apply the oils to a bandage with an eye dropper and tape securely to the site. Leave on for several hours or overnight. Carefully remove the bandage and withdraw the splinter.

GET IT OUT BANDAGE

Try a bandage of this blend on your splinter for its drawing properties, including analgesic, antibacterial, anti-inflammatory, antiseptic, bactericidal, and cicatrisant ingredients, which bring about healing quickly once that splinter is out.

YIELD: 1 APPLICATION

1 drop myrrh oil
1 drop geranium oil
5 drops carrier oil

Mix the ingredients well. Apply a few drops of the mixture to a bandage or a piece of gauze and secure to the site. Leave on for several hours or overnight. Carefully remove the bandage and withdraw the splinter.

SPRAIN

One wrong move can cause us to stretch our ligaments and create a sprain in our muscles and tendons. Seek medical attention and keep the affected area still. While in recovery, essential oils can reduce the swelling and pain.

Essential Oils: lavender, ginger, helichrysum, eucalyptus, clove, thyme, marjoram, rosemary, birch, vetiver, pine, black pepper, jasmine, camphor, frankincense, cypress, cinnamon, wintergreen, white fir, melissa, jasmine, and chamomile

KASSIE'S SPRAIN BATH SALTS

This bath salts recipe has the essential oils needed to reduce swelling and inflammation and relieve pain, and will make your skin baby-soft to boot! The therapeutic properties in this blend contain analgesic, antispasmodic, and anti-inflammatory agents.

Yield: 5 to 6 applications

7 drops white fir oil
7 drops rosemary oil
7 drops marjoram oil
1 ounce carrier oil
3 cups salts (pink Himalayan salt, sea salt, Epsom salts)
1 tablespoon milk (optional for adults, recommended for children)

Add the oils to the salt. Stir until the mixture is well blended. Put in a jar with a lid. Let sit for 24 hours and stir again. Do not make the bathwater too hot, as the oils will dissipate. Do not add the salts when the water is running, but add ½ cup of the bath salt mixture and the milk to the water as you get into the tub. Oftentimes people add 1 tablespoon milk to the water; this will cause the essential oil to blend into the water and not float on top. Store the remainder in a jar with a tight-fitting lid, in a cool, dark area, for up to 3 months.

REMI'S SPRAIN POULTICE

This pain-reducing poultice is full of essential oils that will speed up the healing process and help you on your road to recovery. This recipe has antispasmodic, anti-inflammatory, anti-rheumatic, and analgesic elements.

Yield: 1 application

3 drops lavender oil
1 drop marjoram oil
1 drop camphor oil
1 wet cloth

Using an eye dropper, drip the oils onto a damp, warm cloth. Apply the cloth to the affected area as often as desired. Change when the cloth becomes uncomfortable.

JAKE'S RUB

This rub will help reduce swelling and contains pain-relieving essential oils that will get you back on your feet quickly. The components of this blend include analgesic, antispasmodic, antiarthritic, anti-inflammatory, and antispasmodic properties.

Yield: 4 to 10 applications

3 drops thyme oil
3 drops ginger oil
2 drops jasmine oil
1 drop black pepper oil
2 ounces carrier oil

In a small container, drip the essential oils. Pour

in the carrier oil and swirl to mix the oils. Rub the sprained area lightly with your fingertips or a soft cloth dipped into the mixture to ensure that the essential oils are distributed over the skin. You can also pour into a roll-on bottle and roll onto the desired area. Be sure not to get any into the eyes or sensitive areas. Store the remainder in a jar with a tight-fitting lid, in a cool, dark area, for up to 3 months.

STRESS

Stress can cause illness, disease, and a loss of social and family life. We are all constantly on the lookout for ways to reduce our stress. In today's crazy and hectic world, it is easy to feel pushed to the breaking point. Essential oils can play a huge part in minimizing that overwhelmed and overworked feeling and promote a sense of well-being and peace.

Essential Oils: peppermint, frankincense, petitgrain, helichrysum, melissa, cassia, cedarwood, lavender, bergamot, chamomile, lemon, marjoram, neroli, sandalwood, thyme, rosemary, grapefruit, basil, patchouli, clary sage, vetiver, cardamom, benzoin, pine, rose, ylang-ylang, spikenard, spearmint, cinnamon, cypress, and geranium

MURF'S STRESS-FREE POWDER

Don't worry about it! When you want to have a good night's sleep without stressing about anything, this calming, sleep-inducing remedy will be perfect for you. Let the essential oils work their magic so that your mind can relax while you drift off to slumber with the help of their antidepressant, nervine, and sedative properties.

Yield: 10 to 20 applications

3 drops geranium oil
3 drops chamomile oil
3 drops vetiver oil
¼ cup cornstarch

Combine the ingredients very well with a whisk. Pour into a mason jar with holes poked into the lid. Shake the powder inside a pillowcase or under the sheets, and wake up in the morning with renewed energy after a cool, peaceful night's sleep. When storing your jar, you can place a piece of plastic wrap under the lid so that the powder won't spill out of the jar. Store in a jar with a tight-fitting lid, in a cool, dark, dry area, for up to 3 months.

LAST THING I DO BATH SALTS

This nighttime recipe for your bath will have you yawning and smiling at the same time as it relieves your stress and calms those frantic nerves. Its pleasant aroma and antidepressant, antispasmodic, nervine, sedative, and hypotensive properties will have you relaxing in no time.

Yield: 5 to 6 applications

5 drops rose oil
5 drops patchouli oil
5 drops clary sage oil
5 drops lavender oil
1 ounce carrier oil
3 cups salts (pink Himalayan salt, sea salt,
    Epsom salts)
1 tablespoon milk (optional for adults,
    recommended for children)

Add the oils to the salt. Stir until the mixture is well blended. Put in a jar with a lid. Let sit for 24 hours and stir again. Do not make the bathwater too hot, as the oils will dissipate. Do not add the salts when the water is running, but add ½ cup of the bath salt mixture and the milk to the water as you get into the tub. Oftentimes people add 1 tablespoon milk to the water; this will cause the essential oil to blend into the water and not float on top. Store the remainder in a jar with a tight-fitting lid, in a cool, dark area, for up to 3 months.

KICK-ASS DIFFUSER

This is a powerful diffuse recipe that uses the essential oils best known for their stress-reducing benefits. It packs a punch as it delivers the sedative, tranquilizing, antidepressant, and nervine properties right to your brain and soul. Your stress level will sink lower and lower as you take in this aromatic blend.

Yield: 1 application

3 drops vetiver oil
2 drops rosemary oil
2 drops basil oil
2 drops clary sage oil
Water

Most diffusers come with directions for using essential oils. Add the manufacturer's recommended amount of water and the oils to the diffuser and run your delightful diffuser several times a day to receive the desired effect.

STRETCH MARKS

Pregnancy is a wonderful time for many women, but its aftereffects—those pink scars that develop on the stomach or thighs during rapid weight gain—are not so wonderful. These marks can be reduced dramatically with the assistance of essential oils.

Essential Oils: lavender, frankincense, grapefruit, helichrysum, sandalwood, ylang-ylang, cypress, and jasmine

STRETCH MARK OIL

This recipe uses essential oils that can reduce stretch marks, scarring, and discoloration. Use daily until desired results are achieved. A few of the healing ingredients in this blend include anti-inflammatory, astringent, cicatrisant, and cytophylactic properties.

YIELD: 4 TO 10 APPLICATIONS

2 drops helichrysum oil
2 drops lavender oil
2 drops geranium oil
2 drops frankincense oil
2 ounces melted coconut oil

In a small container, drip the essential oils. Pour in the coconut oil and swirl to mix the oils. Rub the stretch mark area lightly with your fingertips or a soft cloth dipped into the mixture to ensure that the essential oils are distributed over the skin. You can also pour into a roll-on bottle and roll onto the desired area. Be sure not to get any into the eyes or sensitive areas. Store the remainder in a jar with a tight-fitting lid, in a cool, dark area, for up to 3 months.

RUB-A-DUB-DUB

Apply this rub at bedtime and let these essential oils lighten and smooth those stretch marks all night long with the added benefit of getting a good night's sleep. The properties at work here include astringent, stimulant, antiseptic, cicatrisant, and tissue-regeneration elements.

YIELD: 2 TO 6 APPLICATIONS

4 drops grapefruit oil
1 drop lavender oil
1 drop helichrysum oil
1 ounce carrier oil

In a small container, drip the essential oils. Pour in the carrier oil and swirl to mix the oils. Rub the desired area lightly with your fingertips or a soft cloth dipped into the mixture to ensure that the essential oils are distributed over the skin. You can also pour into a roll-on bottle and roll onto the desired area. Be sure not to get any into the eyes or sensitive areas. Store unused portion in a jar with a tight-fitting lid, in a cool, dark area, for up to 3 months.

STYE

Characterized by small red bumps that are painful to the touch, a stye is an infection of the sweat glands, usually on the eyelid. When on the lash line, blinking can be painful and uncomfortable—like you have a sticker in your eye. Essential oils can bring relief and have been known to even eradicate styes. Never place essential oils directly in or on the eye.

Essential Oils: lavender, chamomile, frankincense, helichrysum, and tea tree (melaleuca)

HURTS LIKE HELL EYE RUB

Roll this recipe full of healing essential oils around the eye area, but never directly onto the eyeball. The healing properties include analgesic, anti-inflammatory, antiseptic, and cicatrisant properties and will turn that painful stye into a barely noticeable bump.

Yield: 1 application

2 drops frankincense oil
1 drop tea tree (melaleuca) oil
1 drop chamomile oil
1 teaspoon carrier oil

In a small container, drip the essential oils. Pour in the carrier oil and swirl to mix the oils. Rub the stye area lightly with your fingertips or a soft cloth dipped into the mixture to ensure that the essential oils are distributed over the skin, but make sure you don't get any onto the eyeball itself. You can also pour into a roll-on bottle and roll onto the desired area. Be sure not to get any into the eyes or sensitive areas. If any of the mixture remains, store in a container with a tight-fitting lid in the refrigerator for up to 3 days.

STYE EYE COMPRESS

This cool compress will feel so good instantly and begin healing that stye with its antiseptic, anti-inflammatory, antiviral, cicatrisant, and tonic properties as well as tissue-regeneration elements.

Yield: 2 to 6 applications

2 drops tea tree (melaleuca) oil
1 drop lavender oil
1 drop helichrysum oil
1 ounce carrier oil

Mix the ingredients together. Apply to a clean cloth and lay the cloth over the closed eye. Never let essential oils get onto the actual eyeball. Let sit for 10 to 15 minutes or until uncomfortable. Reapply as needed. Store unused portion in a jar with a tight-fitting lid, in a cool, dark area, for up to 3 months.

SUNBURN

Who hasn't spent a day outside in the glorious sun, only to end up with red, painful skin that soon begins to peel off? A sunburn consists of a reddening of the outer layer of skin by too much sun, which causes heat and pain. There are many essential oils that can bring relief and lessen the effects of sunburn. If blisters are present, seek medical attention. Severe sunburns in children are a medical emergency. In our lifetime, protecting yourself from the sun has become a life or death practice due to the rise of skin cancer. Always wear sunscreen!

Essential Oils: lavender, peppermint, chamomile, tea tree (melaleuca), geranium, marjoram, rose, frankincense, and sandalwood

RED OUT WASH

This wash contains essential oils that will speed the healing of your sunburn and bring immediate relief. The healing properties in this recipe include analgesic, anti-inflammatory, antiseptic, cicatrisant, and cytophylactic agents.

Yield: 1 application

4 drops lavender oil
4 drops peppermint oil
3 drops frankincense oil
1 bowl room-temperature water

Combine the oils with the water in the bowl. With a soft washcloth, apply the mixture to the affected area and let air dry. Never apply to open wounds or near sensitive body parts.

SUNBURN SPRAY

Keep a bottle of this handy in the summertime to bring instant relief to your guests and friends when they have a little too much outdoor fun. The skin healing properties include antibiotic, anti-inflammatory, antiseptic, cicatrisant, and immune-stimulating components.

Yield: 50 to 100 sprays per 4-ounce bottle

6 drops lavender oil
5 drops tea tree (melaleuca) oil
4 drops chamomile oil

1 drop sandalwood oil
1 tablespoon vinegar
4 ounces water

Combine the ingredients in a 4-ounce spray bottle and lightly spray the affected area. Allow to air dry. The essential oils will be absorbed into the skin by contact. Store in the spray bottle in a cool, dark area for up to 3 months.

COOLING BATH

When your body feels like it's on fire from your sunburn, this bath feels like it is sucking the heat right out of you. The essential oils in this recipe have therapeutic properties that enable them to assist with healing burns and provide pain-reducing results with their antiseptic, astringent, cicatrisant, and tonic properties.

Yield: 1 application

4 drops geranium oil
4 drops marjoram oil
3 drops rose oil
1 tablespoon carrier oil
1 tablespoon milk (optional for adults,
　　recommended for children)

While the bathwater is running, pour the ingredients into the bath. Make sure that the water is not so hot as to cause the essential oils to dissipate. Oftentimes people add 1 tablespoon milk

to the water; this will cause the essential oil to blend into the water and not float on top. Soak in the water as long as you are comfortable.

TENDONITIS

The tendons surrounding the joints become inflamed and can cause severe pain for various reasons. My father has suffered from tendonitis for years and gets great relief from the recipes below. Essential oils can reduce pain, swelling, and the severity of this disease.

Essential Oils: wintergreen, birch, basil, peppermint, oregano, helichrysum, cypress, lavender, lemon, lemongrass, and grapefruit

TENDON BATH SALTS

These essential oils will work with the salts to assist with healing and relieving pain. The ingredients in this blend include antispasmodic, anti-inflammatory, tissue-regeneration, nervine, and sedative properties.

Yield: 5 to 6 applications

7 drops helichrysum oil

7 drops grapefruit oil

7 drops lemongrass oil

1 ounce carrier oil

3 cups salts (pink Himalayan salt, sea salt, Epsom salts)

1 tablespoon milk (optional for adults, recommended for children)

Add the oils to the salt. Stir until the mixture is well blended. Put in a jar with a lid. Let sit for 24 hours and stir again. Do not make the bathwater too hot, as the oils will dissipate. Do not add the salts when the water is running, but add ½ cup of the bath salt mixture and the milk to the water as you get into the tub. Oftentimes people add 1 tablespoon milk to the water; this will cause the essential oil to blend into the water and not float on top. Store the remainder in a jar with a tight-fitting lid, in a cool, dark area, for up to 3 months.

JOINT RUB

This is a great rub to use at nighttime to bring relief to sore tendons. These essential oils have the therapeutic properties you need to begin the healing process, such as anti-inflammatory, nervine, sedative, analgesic, and anesthetic elements.

Yield: 2 to 6 applications

2 drops lemongrass oil

2 drops peppermint oil

2 drops cypress oil

1 ounce carrier oil

In a small container, drip the essential oils. Pour in the carrier oil and swirl to mix the oils. Rub the sore tendon area lightly with your fingertips or a soft cloth dipped into the mixture to ensure that the essential oils are distributed over the skin. You can also pour into a roll-on bottle and roll onto the desired area. Be sure not to get any into the eyes or sensitive areas. Store unused portion in a jar with a tight-fitting lid, in a cool, dark area, for up to 3 months.

PAIN WRAP

This is a great wrap to use before going out to be active. The healing properties of these essential oils will help you get back in the game. A few of the components in this recipe include anti-inflammatory, antispasmodic, tissue regeneration, and analgesic properties.

Yield: 2 to 6 applications

3 drops helichrysum oil

2 drops lavender oil

2 drops basil oil

1 ounce carrier oil

Mix the ingredients and apply about a teaspoon

of the mixture to a long piece of muslin or cotton. Wrap the treated material around the wrist, knee, ankle, or other affected area. Leave for at least 15 minutes. Store unused portion in a jar with a tight-fitting lid, in a cool, dark area, for up to 3 months.

THYROID

This gland can be responsible for a wide variety of ailments in the body. My daughter has been on thyroid medication to bring her thyroid back into balance. She no longer takes the medication, but if she is feeling out of sorts, she will use this recipe to feel better. If your doctor has diagnosed you with a thyroid condition, essential oils can help to regulate the thyroid and get your body back in balance.

Essential Oils: melissa, vetiver, peppermint, lemon, lime, grapefruit, orange, wild orange, myrrh, frankincense, cedarwood, sandalwood, and geranium

THYROID SPRAY

These essential oils are derived from plants that have been used for thousands of years to regulate the thyroid. The therapeutic properties that help to support the endocrine system include nervine, anti-inflammatory, circulatory, immune-stimulant, tonic, and detoxifying elements.

YIELD: 50 TO 100 SPRAYS PER 4-OUNCE BOTTLE

3 drops geranium oil
3 drops myrrh oil
3 drops peppermint oil
3 drops frankincense oil
3 drops lemon oil
4 ounces water

Combine the ingredients in a 4-ounce spray bottle and lightly spray the affected area. Allow to air dry. The essential oils will be absorbed into the skin by contact or by the lungs if sprayed into the air. You can also diffuse this same recipe. Store in the spray bottle in a cool, dark area for up to 3 months.

TINNITUS

A sound or ringing in the ear when no actual sound is being made. Tinnitus can be annoying at best, and cause lack of sleep when it appears at night. Essential oils rubbed on the outer ear can help relieve this uncomfortable condition. Never put essential oils directly into the ear canal.

Essential Oils: lavender, peppermint, basil, frankincense, helichrysum, spearmint, sandalwood, rosemary, geranium, and cypress

DAMN RINGING COMPRESS!

These essential oils can put an end to that blasted ringing! The properties at work here contain anticoagulant, anti-inflammatory, and antispasmodic elements.

YIELD: 2 TO 6 APPLICATIONS

2 drops lavender oil
2 drops spearmint oil
2 drops helichrysum oil
1 ounce carrier oil

Mix the ingredients together and pour a small amount onto a small cloth or cotton ball. Apply the cloth to area desired as often as needed.

Never put essential oils directly inside the ear. Store unused portion in a jar with a tight-fitting lid, in a cool, dark area, for up to 3 months.

OUTER EAR MASSAGE

I have actually been woken up out of a dead sleep with ringing in my ears. I keep a little bottle of this by my bed to rub on my outer ear when it just becomes too much. The ring-reducing elements in these oils are analgesic, anti-inflammatory, sedative, and antispasmodic properties.

YIELD: 2 TO 6 APPLICATIONS

3 drops sandalwood oil
3 drops geranium oil
2 drops basil oil
2 drops frankincense oil
1 ounce carrier oil

In a small container, drip the essential oils. Pour in the carrier oil and swirl to mix the oils. Rub the outer ear area lightly with your fingertips or a soft cloth dipped into the mixture to ensure that the essential oils are distributed over the skin. You can also pour into a roll-on bottle and roll onto the desired area. Be sure not to get any into the eyes or sensitive areas. Store unused portion in a jar with a tight-fitting lid, in a cool, dark area, for up to 3 months.

TONSILLITIS

The tonsils are two small glands on the interior sides of the throat. These can become swollen for a myriad of reasons: strep, virus, bacteria, colds, and so on. Many people have their tonsils removed if the inflammation becomes chronic, so seek medical attention if this is the case. I spent two weeks every year when I was a teenager with painful tonsillitis. Gargling with saltwater often helps reduce some of the pain. These essential oils have been distilled from plants and herbs that were used for centuries to relieve tonsillitis and other throat issues.

Essential Oils: clove, cinnamon, ginger, lemongrass, lavender, frankincense, lemon, marjoram, oregano, thyme, bergamot, geranium, and Roman chamomile

POWERFUL GARGLE

This recipe is the ultimate throat-soothing gargle. These essential oils will work wonders and have you feeling great in no time with their antibacterial, cooling, analgesic, anti-inflammatory, and antiviral properties.

Yield: 1 to 2 applications

2 drops cinnamon oil

2 drops lemongrass oil

2 drops clove oil

4 ounces water

Ensure that your essential oils are safe for consumption and internal use and are clinical/therapeutic grade. Combine the oils and water in a glass. Put a small amount into your mouth and rapidly swish around. Spit it all out when done. Store unused portion in a jar with a tight-fitting lid, in a cool, dark area or the refrigerator, for up to 1 day.

THROAT RUB

We don't realize how much we swallow until we have a sore throat. End the pain in your throat with this recipe, which will get you through the day or night with its healing properties, some of which are analgesic, antibiotic, anti-infectious, and anti-inflammatory agents.

Yield: 4 to 10 applications

3 drops bergamot oil

3 drops tea tree (melaleuca) oil

3 drops lemongrass oil

3 drops Roman chamomile oil

2 ounces carrier oil

In a small container, drip the essential oils. Pour in the carrier oil and swirl to mix the oils. Rub the outer throat and jaw area lightly with your fingertips or a soft cloth dipped into the mixture to ensure that the essential oils are distributed over the skin. You can also pour into a roll-on bottle and roll onto the desired area. Be sure not to get any into the eyes or sensitive areas. Store the remainder in a jar with a tight-fitting lid, in a cool, dark area, for up to 3 months.

TOOTHACHE

Often when nerves in the teeth are inflamed, a toothache can result and the pain ranges from mild to excruciating. Essential oils rubbed on the gums have helped people deal with this pain and also reduce inflammation. If swelling is present, or if pain is chronic or severe, you must see a dentist.

Essential Oils: thieves', chamomile, clove, peppermint, spearmint, tea tree (melaleuca), hyssop, cinnamon, cajeput, lemon, and myrrh

ADULT TOOTH RELIEVER

This is a powerful remedy that works instantaneously. This is what I use when I have a toothache due to the analgesic, anti-inflammatory, antiseptic, dental-pain-relieving, and sedative properties.

YIELD: 1 APPLICATION

4 drops clove oil
1 drop orange oil
1 teaspoon carrier oil

Ensure that your essential oil is safe for consumption and internal use and is clinical/therapeutic grade. Mix the ingredients together and either dab on the toothache with your fingertip, or place on a piece of gauze and hold between the teeth. If any of the mixture remains, store in a container with a tight-fitting lid in the refrigerator for up to 3 days.

CHILD TOOTH RELIEVER

Children, whose teeth are developing, often suffer from all sorts of tooth-related problems. This is a safe way to get them fast results and a good night's sleep at the same time. The pain-relieving elements of this blend contain anti-inflammatory, antiseptic, and sedative properties. Do not use essential oils on any child under the age of four.

YIELD: 1 APPLICATION

3 drops chamomile oil
1 drop orange oil
1 teaspoon carrier oil

Ensure that your essential oil is safe for consumption and internal use and is clinical/therapeutic grade. Mix the ingredients together and either dab on the toothache with your fingertip, or place on a piece of gauze and hold between the teeth. If any of the mixture remains, store in a container with a tight-fitting lid in the refrigerator for up to 3 days.

TOOTHACHE OIL PULL

This old-time remedy is a quick and safe way to get relief from the pounding, throbbing pain of a toothache. These oils contain analgesic, anesthetic, anti-infectious, anti-inflammatory, and sedative properties.

YIELD: 1 APPLICATION

2 drops clove oil
2 drops peppermint oil
1 teaspoon carrier oil

Ensure that your essential oils are safe for consumption and internal use and are clinical/therapeutic grade. Mix the ingredients well and swish through the teeth and mouth for 5 minutes, then spit out. Do not swallow.

ULCERS (MOUTH)

A common occurrence in many individuals, mouth ulcers are painful and can recur sometimes for no known reason. A doctor can diagnose an ulcer versus something more serious, so it's best to get a professional diagnosis for any types of mouth sore. Essential oils can alleviate the pain associated with mouth ulcers and help to heal them.

Essential Oils: lemon, geranium, peppermint, tangerine, tea tree (melaleuca), orange, myrrh, lime, cypress, clary sage, bergamot, Roman chamomile, oregano, fennel, thyme, frankincense, lemongrass, basil, and clove

BODY ULCER POULTICE

These essential oils have long been used to treat ulcers on the body. Their healing properties work fast and effectively to heal that ulcer and get you back to normal. The healing and pain-relieving properties in this blend include antibacterial, antibiotic, anti-infectious, anti-inflammatory, antimicrobial, antiseptic, and cicatrisant elements.

YIELD: 1 APPLICATION

2 drops tea tree (melaleuca) oil

2 drops frankincense oil

2 drops geranium oil

1 tablespoon carrier oil

1 wet cloth

Mix the ingredients together in a small container. Pour onto a wet, warm cloth and apply the cloth to the affected area; let sit for 10 to 20 minutes. Do this 3 times daily until the ulcer improves. Change as the cloth temperature becomes uncomfortable.

MOUTH ULCER SWISHER

This recipe burns a little, but the pain is worth it when you see how fast your mouth ulcer will heal. The healing and pain-relieving properties in this recipe are, in part, analgesic, anesthetic, anti-infectious, and anti-inflammatory.

Yield: 1 to 2 applications

2 drops peppermint oil

2 drops thyme oil

2 drops lemon oil

2 drops tea tree (melaleuca) oil

1 ounce vodka or brandy

1 ounce water

Ensure that your essential oil is safe for consumption and internal use and is clinical/therapeutic grade. Combine the oils, water, and vodka or brandy in a glass. Put a small amount into your mouth and rapidly swish around. Spit it all out when done (do not swallow). Repeat as needed. Store any remainder in a jar with a tight-fitting lid, in the refrigerator or a cool, dark area, for up to 24 hours.

NEAT ULCER APPLICATION

Tea tree oil is a true wonder in the essential oil world. Its healing properties are amazingly diverse and some of them include antibacterial, antibiotic, anti-infectious, anti-inflammatory, antimicrobial, antiseptic, and cicatrisant elements.

Yield: 1 applications

1 drop tea tree (melaleuca) oil

A few essential oils can be placed directly on the skin (neat) without adding carrier oil to them. Be sure that you are using a safe and pure essential oil before placing on the body, as essential oils can be very powerful. Dab the oil onto the ulcer and repeat as needed.

VAGINAL ITCH

There are a variety of causes for an itch in the vaginal area, most of which are easily treatable. Essential oils can be used to stop the itching, but if it's chronic, it is important to seek a medical diagnosis. Never put essential oils directly on your genitals.

Essential Oils: bergamot, tea tree (melaleuca), myrrh, lavender, and cedarwood

PRIVATE BATH

These gentle, effective essential oils will help you to end that embarrassing itch—and they smell good, too! The healing properties include analgesic, antibiotic, antiseptic, and vulnerary agents.

YIELD: 1 APPLICATION

3 drops bergamot oil
3 drops lavender oil
2 drops cedarwood oil
2 drops myrrh oil
3 drops tea tree (melaleuca) oil
1 tablespoon carrier oil
1 tablespoon milk (optional for adults, recommended for children)

While the bathwater is running, pour the ingredients into the bath. Make sure that the water is not so hot as to cause the essential oils to dissipate. Oftentimes people add 1 tablespoon milk to the water; this will cause the essential oil to blend into the water and not float on top. Soak in the water as long as you are comfortable.

VARICOSE VEINS

Women have long used essential oils to not only soften the look of varicose veins, but also to reduce the swelling that can occur when standing for long periods of time. Never massage a varicose vein with too much pressure. A light, gentle stroke is all you need for this condition; too much pressure can cause a rupture in the vein.

Essential Oils: cypress, juniper berry, lavender, lemon, orange, grapefruit, geranium, rosemary, lemongrass, peppermint, myrrh, frankincense, chamomile, and helichrysum

VEIN COMPRESS

Apply this compress while you rest and you will be amazed how the pain-reducing, vein-reducing, therapeutic properties of these essential oils work. A few of these are analgesic, anti-inflammatory, antineuralgic, antispasmodic, cooling, nervine, and sedative.

YIELD: 2 TO 6 APPLICATIONS

4 drops chamomile oil
4 drops lavender oil
2 drops frankincense oil
1 ounce carrier oil
1 wet cloth

Mix the ingredients together in a small container. Dab a wet, warm cloth into the mixture and apply the cloth lightly to the vein area as often as needed. Change as cloth temperature becomes uncomfortable. Store unused portion in a jar with a tight-fitting lid, in a cool, dark area, for up to 3 months.

VAIN VEIN

This recipe can reduce the appearance of varicose veins and also help shrink them. The healing elements of this recipe include anti-inflammatory, vasoconstrictor, antispasmodic, and restorative properties.

YIELD: 2 TO 6 APPLICATIONS

4 drops lavender oil
4 drops cypress oil
2 drops lemongrass oil

1 ounce carrier oil

Mix the ingredients together in a small container. Apply to a cloth and lay the cloth on the affected area as often as needed. Do not rub or apply pressure. Store unused portion in a jar with a tight-fitting lid, in a cool, dark area, for up to 3 months.

I WANNA WEAR SHORT-SHORTS BATH

It's summertime and that means shorts and skirts. Get rid of those unsightly blue veins with this healing remedy. The therapeutic properties in this blend contain anti-inflammatory, analgesic, antispasmodic, antibruising, and anticoagulant components.

YIELD: 1 APPLICATION

2 drops lemon oil
2 drops grapefruit oil
2 drops helichrysum oil
2 drops frankincense oil
2 drops lavender oil
1 tablespoon carrier oil
1 tablespoon milk (optional for adults, recommended for children)

While the bathwater is running, pour the ingredients into the bath. Make sure that the water is not so hot as to cause the essential oils to dissi-

pate. Oftentimes people add 1 tablespoon milk to the water; this will cause the essential oil to blend into the water and not float on top. Soak in the water as long as you are comfortable.

VERTIGO

Vertigo is a dizzy, nauseated feeling that can strike for apparently no reason. I had a friend that suffered from this ailment, and she would start getting very unbalanced at the most inopportune times. This was a sad and embarrassing condition for her. These recipes helped with bringing her some control and relieved a lot of the stress she had about vertigo. Essential oils can help calm and balance your system and reduce the effects of vertigo.

Essential Oils: lavender, peppermint, melissa, frankincense, ginger, ylang-ylang, basil, geranium, helichrysum, Roman chamomile, thyme, and rosemary

STOP THE NAUSEA DRINK

This is the go-to essential oil for nausea and stomach issues. Ginger works effectively and quickly with its analgesic, antiemetic, antispasmodic, and stomachic properties.

YIELD: 1 TO 2 APPLICATIONS

1 drop ginger oil
2 to 4 ounces water

Drip the ginger oil into a glass of water and drink slowly. Store unused portion in a jar with a tight-fitting lid, in a cool, dark area or the refrigerator, for up to 1 day.

DIZZY RUB

The essential oils in this recipe have long been used to reduce that swimming, dizzy feeling that accompanies vertigo. The healing and balancing properties in this blend contain analgesic, carminative, emmenagogue, tonic, antispasmodic, cephalic, and stimulating agents.

YIELD: 1 APPLICATION

1 drop frankincense oil
1 drop peppermint oil
1 teaspoon carrier oil

In a small container, drip the essential oils. Pour in the carrier oil and swirl to mix the oils. Rub the desired area lightly with your fingertips or a soft cloth dipped into the mixture to ensure that the essential oils are distributed over the skin. You can also pour into a roll-on bottle and roll onto the desired area. Be sure not to get any into the eyes or sensitive areas. If any of the mixture remains, store in a container with a tight-fitting lid in the refrigerator for up to 3 days.

INHALE

Carry a vial of these therapeutic essential oils with you and when that uncomfortable feeling begins to descend, take a sniff from your vial and you will feel better quickly. Each of these oils contains, in part, analgesic, anti-inflammatory, restorative, and uplifting properties.

Yield: 1 application

1 drop peppermint oil, or 1 drop lavender oil

Place the drop of essential oil on a handkerchief or tissue, in the palm of your hand, or in an essential oil inhaler. Cup to your nose and inhale the aroma. Repeat several times daily or as needed.

VIRAL INFECTION

Essential oils not only help with the pain, nausea, and discomfort of a viral infection, but can actually protect a person's surroundings so that the virus cannot survive to be passed to anyone else. Viral infections are very contagious, and a good way to protect your family is to begin using essential oils in the home once you know a virus has found its way to your town. If symptoms do develop, seek medical attention.

Essential Oils: peppermint, sandalwood, basil, cassia, tea tree (melaleuca), melissa, myrrh, cajeput, lime, grapefruit, clary sage, thyme, oregano, cinnamon, clove, eucalyptus, frankincense, helichrysum, lemon, lemongrass, and marjoram

VIRAL ROOM SPRAY

The therapeutic properties of these essential oils disinfect and keep your room, car, office space, and home free of airborne germs that can spread viruses. The healing and protecting components in this recipe are analgesic, antifungal, anti-infectious, anti-inflammatory, antiseptic, and antimicrobial properties.

Yield: 50 to 100 sprays per 4-ounce bottle

5 drops peppermint oil

5 drops lime oil

3 drops clove oil

5 drops lemon oil

4 ounces water

Combine the ingredients in a 4-ounce spray bottle and lightly spray the room area. Allow to air dry. These oils have germ-fighting properties to assist in keeping your home virus free. Store in the spray bottle in a cool, dark area for up to 3 months.

VIRAL BODY SPRAY

A spray of this in the morning keeps you smelling fresh, but secretly protects you all day from virus-spreading germs. A few of the protecting elements in this recipe are analgesic, antibacterial, anti-inflammatory, antimicrobial, antiseptic, and antiviral agents.

YIELD: 50 TO 100 SPRAYS PER 4-OUNCE BOTTLE

3 drops sandalwood oil

3 drops myrrh oil

3 drops melissa oil

3 drops eucalyptus oil

4 ounces water

Combine the ingredients in a 4-ounce spray bottle and lightly spray the affected area. Allow to air dry. The essential oils will be absorbed into the skin by contact or by the lungs if sprayed into the air. Store in the spray bottle in a cool, dark area for up to 3 months.

CLEAN THE AIR

This diffuser keeps your home smelling fresh while the essential oils fight the viral germs that run rampant during certain times of the year. The protecting elements include astringent, detoxifier, antiseptic, antispasmodic, antiviral, bactericidal, and cephalic components.

YIELD: 1 APPLICATION

3 drops marjoram oil

3 drops lemon oil

3 drops eucalyptus oil

Water

Most diffusers come with directions for using essential oils. Add the manufacturer's recommended amount of water and the oils to the diffuser and run your delightful diffuser several times a day to receive the desired effect.

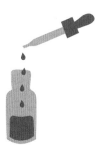

WARTS

There are several types of warts, which are usually harmless and can last from months to years, but they are also often ugly. The essential oils that come from plants and herbs are one of the ways in which warts have been eradicated for centuries. But warts can always make a sneaky comeback, so you may have to repeat these steps to end them for good!

Essential Oils: tea tree (melaleuca), lemon, oregano, lime, cinnamon, thyme, cypress, cajeput, and clove

WART-REMOVER RUB

My sister used this recipe daily on her grandson's wart, and after a week or two it just shriveled up and died. It's very effective. The healing components of this blend include astringent, detoxifier, antibacterial, antifungal, fungicide, anti-infectious, and antiviral properties.

YIELD: 1 TO 2 APPLICATIONS

2 drops tea tree (melaleuca) oil
2 drops lemon oil
2 drops cajeput oil
1 tablespoon carrier oil

In a small container, drip the essential oils. Pour in the carrier oil and swirl to mix the oils. Rub the wart lightly with your fingertips or a soft cloth dipped into the mixture to ensure that the essential oils are distributed over the skin. You can also pour into a roll-on bottle and roll onto the desired area. Be sure not to get any into the eyes or sensitive areas. Apply several times a day until the wart falls off or disappears. Store the remainder in a jar with a tight-fitting lid, in a cool, dark area, for up to 1 month.

DAB IT ON

Tea tree oil has long been used as a wart killer with its antibacterial, antibiotic, antifungal, anti-inflammatory, antimicrobial, antiparasitic, and antiviral components, to name a few.

YIELD: 1 APPLICATION

1 drop tea tree (melaleuca) oil

A few essential oils can be placed directly on the skin (neat) without adding carrier oil to them. Be sure that you are using a safe, pure essential oil before placing on the body, as essential oils can be very powerful. Just dab this on your wart and repeat several times a day for 1 to 2 weeks.

WART BANDAGE

This bandage ensures that the essential oils

remain on your wart long enough to let their therapeutic properties seep into your skin and begin the work of killing it off. These essential oils contain, in part, antibacterial, antibiotic, antifungal, anti-inflammatory, antimicrobial, antiparasitic, and antiviral properties.

YIELD: 1 APPLICATION

1 drop tea tree (melaleuca) oil

1 drop lemon oil

4 drops carrier oil

Mix the ingredients well in a small container. Apply a few drops of the ingredients to a bandage or a piece of gauze with an eye dropper and secure to the site. Leave on for several hours or overnight. Repeat daily until the wart is gone.

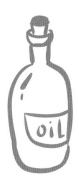

WITHDRAWAL
(Drugs, Alcohol, and Tobacco)

Withdrawing from drugs, alcohol, or tobacco can be a heart-wrenching ordeal. The person not only experiences physical pain, but mental anguish as well. It's best to have this process monitored by a professional. Essential oils can help a person by relaxing and calming them, helping to eradicate pain, and ridding the room and person of negative thoughts associated with the withdrawal process.

Essential Oils: lavender, lemon, lime, orange, wild orange, sandalwood, grapefruit, and marjoram

NEVER AGAIN POWDER

Strengthen your resolve overnight as you sleep when using these powders under your sheets. These essential oils will improve your slumber while working to steady your will. The healing properties in these oils contain analgesic, anticonvulsive, antidepressant, detoxifying, sedative, and restorative elements.

YIELD: 10 TO 20 APPLICATIONS

3 drops lavender oil

3 drops sandalwood oil

3 drops marjoram oil

¼ cup cornstarch

Combine the ingredients very well with a whisk. Pour into a mason jar with holes poked into the lid. Shake the powder inside a pillowcase or under the sheets, and wake up in the morning with renewed energy after a cool, peaceful night's sleep. When storing your jar, you can place a piece of plastic wrap under the lid so that the powder won't spill out of the jar. Store in a jar with a tight-fitting lid, in a cool, dark, dry area, for up to 3 months.

BREAK THE HABIT BATH SALTS

This luxurious bath will help increase your willpower, and the essential oils have long been reported to make withdrawal just a little bit easier. The benefits of these oils include restorative, tonic, analgesic, cephalic, sedative, cordial, and hypotensive properties.

YIELD: 5 TO 6 APPLICATIONS

7 drops wild orange oil

7 drops lime oil

7 drops marjoram oil

1 ounce carrier oil

3 cups salts (pink Himalayan salt, sea salt, Epsom salts)

1 tablespoon milk (optional for adults, recommended for children)

Add the oils to the salt. Stir until the mixture is well blended. Put in a jar with a lid. Let sit for 24 hours and stir again. Do not make the bathwater too hot, as the oils will dissipate. Do not add the salts when the water is running, but add ½ cup of the bath salt mixture and the milk to the water as you get into the tub. Oftentimes people add 1 tablespoon milk to the water; this will cause the essential oil to blend into the water and not float on top. Store the remainder in a jar with a tight-fitting lid, in a cool, dark area, for up to 3 months.

RELAX ME

Just when you feel like you're about to make the wrong choice, take a smell of lavender. It can help relax you to the point that you can hold out just a little bit longer due to its analgesic, antidepressant, detoxifying, sedative, and restorative properties. Lavender can also help relieve irritability and nervous tension.

YIELD: 1 APPLICATION

1 drop lavender oil

Place the drop of essential oil on a handkerchief or tissue, in the palm of your hand, or in an essential oil inhaler. Cup to your nose and inhale the aroma. Repeat several times daily or as needed.

WOUNDS

Small cuts and abrasions can benefit greatly from applying a mixture containing essential oils to the wound. Larger wounds that are gaping, or through several layers of skin, should never be treated with essential oils, but treated instead by a physician. Centuries ago, herbs and plants were the only treatment available for many types of wounds, and they were used with great success. The essential oils we have are the very essence of those plants and herbs. Today the risk of infection can be treated in other ways, but many people prefer the nonchemical-based healing of essential oils.

Essential Oils: lavender, tea tree (melaleuca), frankincense, helichrysum, myrrh, geranium, bergamot, lemon, benzoin, chamomile, clove, cypress, eucalyptus, juniper, niaouli, patchouli, vetiver, and St. John's wort

WOUND WASH

This powerful little recipe is full of healing benefits with its infection and inflammation fighters; this recipe will have your wound healing quickly. The healing agents in this recipe are, in part, antibacterial, antibiotic, antifungal, anti-infectious, anti-inflammatory, antimicrobial, antiparasitic, antiseptic, antiviral, and cicatrisant properties.

YIELD: SEVERAL APPLICATIONS (USE ALL WITHIN ONE DAY; COVER THE BOWL OF INGREDIENTS WITH A TOWEL WHEN NOT IN USE)

5 drops lavender oil
2 drops tea tree (melaleuca) oil
1 drop helichrysum oil
2 ounces room-temperature water

Combine the ingredients in a bowl. With a soft cloth, apply the mixture to the area desired and let air dry. Never apply to an open wound (layers of open skin) or near sensitive body parts.

OUCHIE BANDAGE

This recipe is for a very effective healing bandage that often works magic overnight. The healing benefits include analgesic, antibiotic, antifungal, anti-infectious, and anti-inflammatory elements, to name a few. This is also safe for children over the age of four, but cut the amount of oil in half.

YIELD: 1 APPLICATION

4 drops lavender oil

Apply the oil to a bandage with an eye dropper and tape securely to the site. Leave on for several hours or overnight. Ensure that your oils are therapeutic grade. Certain essential oils, such as lavender, are safe to use "neat" without a carrier oil added.

HEATH'S BOO-BOO BALL

Kids love the Boo-Boo Ball and will ask for it more than anything else when they have a boo-boo. It is very soothing and does not burn or contain any chemicals. Some of the healing and protecting elements in this blend contain anti-bacterial, antibiotic, antifungal, anti-infectious, anti-inflammatory, antimicrobial, antiparasitic, antiseptic, antiviral, and cicatrisant therapeutic properties.

YIELD: 1 APPLICATION

2 drops lavender oil
2 drops tea tree (melaleuca) oil

Place the drops of essential oils on a cotton ball, being careful to not get the oils on your fingers. Place the cotton ball on the area of need and let sit for 15 to 30 minutes, or secure lightly with tape. Repeat throughout the day as needed.

YEAST INFECTION

A fungal infection causing itching, discomfort, and sometimes an odorous discharge, a yeast infection can be an unpleasant event. Never put essential oils in or directly on the genitals, but they can be used in baths to help heal the area and provide a pleasing aroma at the same time. There are many over-the-counter medications today for yeast infections, but many people prefer the old-fashioned, nonchemical, essential oil way.

Essential Oils: lemon and lavender

STOP THE ITCH BATH

Soothing, itch-relieving essential oils help to make you feel better and smell good at the same time. Never apply essential oils directly to the genital area. A few of the healing benefits of these essential oils contain astringent, detoxifying, immune-boosting, analgesic, antibiotic, antifungal, anti-infectious, and anti-inflammatory properties.

YIELD: 1 APPLICATION

7 drops lavender oil

7 drops lemon oil

1 tablespoon carrier oil

*1 tablespoon milk (optional for adults,
   recommended for children)*

While the bathwater is running, pour the ingredients into the bath. Make sure that the water is not so hot as to cause the essential oils to dissipate. Oftentimes people add 1 tablespoon milk to the water; this will cause the essential oil to blend into the water and not float on top. Soak in the water as long as you are comfortable.

YEAST-KILLING DRINK

Lemons have been used for centuries in reducing yeast and fungus growths with their anti-fungal, detoxifying, and astringent properties.

YIELD: 1 TO 2 APPLICATIONS

1 drop lemon oil

2 ounces water

Ensure that your essential oil is safe for consumption and internal use and is clinical/therapeutic grade. Mix the essential oil with the water and drink slowly. Store unused portion in a jar with a tight-fitting lid, in a cool, dark area or the refrigerator, for 1 day.

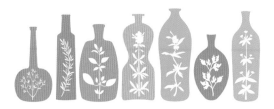

RESOURCES

Earth's Essential Dozen

This is a list of online resources from which you can obtain some of the best essential oils anywhere in the world. I have chosen from all price ranges to give a good selection that you can choose from. You can experiment, read reviews, and research the way that these companies acquire their oils and decide which essential oils are best for you.

1. WWW.FLORIHANA.COM

2. WWW.ELIZABETHVANBUREN.COM

3. WWW.SUNROSEAROMATICS.COM

4. WWW.NATURESGIFT.COM

5. WWW.AV-AT.COM

6. WWW.JADEBLOOM.COM

7. WWW.PIPINGROCK.COM

8. WWW.YOUNGLIVING.COM

9. WWW.DOTERRA.COM

10. WWW.MOUNTAINROSEHERBS.COM

11. WWW.AMEO.COM

12. WWW.NATIVEAMERICANNUTRITIONALS.COM

ACKNOWLEDGMENTS

I wish to thank my husband, Jerry Vance Fite, for supporting me with his patience, interest, kindness, and love during the writing of this book. He had to suffer through a lot of twenty-minute meals when I was on a roll. I love you, Vance.

I would like to thank our families for allowing us to have the many hours that it took to research and compile the countless recipes in this book (and to be test subjects for us more often than they know). We would like to thank our friends for believing in us and for encouraging us to go for our dreams (that especially goes for you, Betsy).

I would like to thank my daughter, Colleen Hoover, who said too many times to "go be it," so I "went and became it," and for giving us the courage to undertake this massive project. Every time I told her I wanted to write this book, she would reply, "So go write it." I am sure that she eventually regretted it because this book is all I've wanted to talk about for over a year now. I love you, Colleen.

I would personally like to thank my daughter, Lin Reynolds, for her thorough research on these essential oils, specifically the "Therapeutic Properties," "Medical Terminology," and

"Fun Facts" sections, and for her time and dedication to this book. Lin and I share so many of the same passions and ideals. She is a true nature's child. I love you, Lin.

I would like to thank Michele Marie Gentles McDaniel for her input, time, research, and the many years we have spent exploring essential oils together. Chele proofread this book and made many corrections. Chele knows what oils are used for which ailments and let me in on too many recipes of hers to count. Chele has joined me on a million adventures involving herbal and essential oil quests. There is not another person on this Earth who I would rather have by my side when conducting research for alternative medicine. We have learned so much together. I love you, Chele.

I would like to thank Clara Daniel for that little bottle of oregano oil when I couldn't shake an illness many years ago. Clara has a passion for essential oils that runs deep and an uncanny ability to know when someone needs them. She is a gifted healer in her own right. If not for her, my love of herbs may never have crossed over to essential oils. Thank you, Clara.

Most of all I would like to thank my mother,

Vannoy Kirkpatrick Gentles, for her unflagging support and her dedication to her children. We love you, Mom. Thanks for supporting us every time we embark on a new quest . . . no matter how crazy it sounds. Every time we call you and say, "Do you want to . . ." you answer, "Yes!" before we even finish our sentence. We love you and Daddy so much.

I would like to thank the people at St. Martin's Press for their desire to take a chance on me and my book. This has been the most exciting endeavor of my life. And a huge thank-you goes to Courtney Littler, my editor, who took a chance on a lady in Texas who loves natural healing. I would also like to thank Liana Krissoff and the entire team at St. Martin's Press for their meticulous editing, assistance, and patience . . . lots of patience.

I would like to thank the amazing team of Dystel & Goderich Literary Management for their support and efforts concerning this book and the entire process. I especially want to thank Jane Dystel for always being accessible to me and answering any questions that I have. Jane, you are the agent that all other agents strive to be. I love you forever.

I want to thank all of the men and women who researched, wrote, and published books, blogs, and Web sites previously about essential oils, because I learned, studied, practiced, and benefitted from every word you wrote, and thousands of other people have benefitted in numerous ways from your work.

A lot of respect goes to all the women and men in the centuries before us who have used plants, herbs, and oils in a quest for a healthier life for themselves and their children. To that first person who took a bite of peppermint when they had a tummy ache, to the person who took a whole acre of lavender flowers and distilled them into a little bottle of potent oil, I thank you.

Vannoy Fite

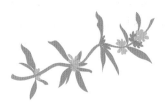

REFERENCES

"25 Uses for Tea Tree (Melaleuca) Oil," *Keeper of the Home* (n.d.). Retrieved August 4, 2014, from http://www.keeperofthehome.org/2013/04/25-uses-for-tea-tree-oil.html.

"All About Herbs, Health, and Wellness," *Herbs Wisdom* (n.d.). Retrieved June 28, 2015, from http://www.herbswisdom.com/.

"Aromatherapy Bible" (n.d.). Retrieved July 2, 2015, from http://aromatherapybible.com/.

"Aura Cacia: 100% Essential Oils" (n.d.). Retrieved July 1, 2015, from http://www.auracacia.com/auracacia/acproducts/acessoils.html.

Dodt, Colleen K. *The Essential Oils Book: Creating Personal Blends for Mind and Body.* Pownal, VT: Storey Communications, 1996.

"Essential Oils," *Buzzle.* Buzzle.com (n.d.). Retrieved September 4, 2014, from http://www.buzzle.com/.

"Essential Oils: Everything You Want and Need to Know" (n.d.). Retrieved July 13, 2014, from http://www.experience-essential-oils.com/.

"Essential Oils," *Oils Information.* Oxford (n.d.). Retrieved August 9, 2013, from http%3A%2F%2Foxford-consultants.tripod.com%2FOilsinformation.htm.

"Essential Oils," *Wikipedia* (n.d.). Retrieved September 6, 2014, from en.wikipedia.org/wiki/Essential oils_ (album).

"Fertility Awareness, Herbal Abortion, and Herbal Contraception," *Fertility Awareness, Herbal Abortion, and Herbal Contraception* (n.d.). Retrieved March 30, 2014, from http://www.sisterzeus.com/.

"Helichrysum Italicum" (n.d.). Retrieved June 29, 2015, from http://helichrysum-italicum.com/.

Keville, Kathi, and Mindy Green. *Aromatherapy: A Complete Guide to the Healing Art.* Berkeley, CA: Crossing, 2009.

Lavabre, Marcel F. *Aromatherapy Workbook.* Rochester, VT: Healing Arts, 1990.

"Lavender: Information About the Different Types of Lavender," *Everything Lavender* (n.d.). Retrieved July 1, 2015, from http://everything-lavender.com/lavender.html.

"Natural Aromatherapy Benefits," *Natural Aromatherapy Benefits* (n.d.). Retrieved July 4, 2014, from http://www.natural-aromatherapy-benefits.com/.

"Organic Facts," *Organic Facts* (n.d.). Retrieved October 1, 2014, from http://www.organicfacts.net/.

Schiller, Carol, and David Schiller. *500 Formulas for Aromatherapy: Mixing Essential Oils for Every Use.* New York: Sterling, 1994.

"Tea Tree Essential Oil Profile, Benefits, and Uses," *Aromaweb* (n.d.). Retrieved July 2, 2015, from http://www.aromaweb.com/essential-oils/tea-tree-oil.asp.

"Tea Tree Oil Uses: 13 Extraordinary Ideas," *Reader's Digest* (n.d.). Retrieved October 3, 2014, from http://www.rd.com/slideshows/tea-tree-oil-uses/.

Walters, Clare. *Aromatherapy: An Illustrated Guide.* Shaftesbury, UK: Element, 1998.

Worwood, Susan E., and Valerie Ann Worwood. *Essential Aromatherapy: A Pocket Guide to Essential Oils and Aromatherapy.* Novato, CA: New World Library, 2003.

INDEX